Incurable and Increasing: The Growing Challenge of Neurodegenerative Diseases

Seusspie

First Printing, 2024

Table of contents

1 Introduction ... 1

1.1 Parkinson's disease ... 2
1.1.1 Different types of Parkinsonian syndromes ... 2
1.1.2 Epidemiology of Parkinson's disease ... 3
1.1.3 Pathophysiology and pathogenesis of Parkinson's disease ... 4
1.1.4 Symptoms and diagnostics of Parkinson's disease ... 7
1.1.5 Treatment of Parkinson's disease ... 10

1.2 Epigenetics ... 12

1.3 miRNA in epigenetic regulation ... 13

1.4 The miRNA cluster 132/212 ... 15
1.4.1 Regulation and effects of miR-132/212 ... 15
1.4.2 miR-132/212 in disease and as therapeutic target ... 19

1.5 Aim of this study ... 22

2 Material ... 23

2.1 Reagents ... 23

2.2 Primers, miRNA mimics and kits ... 24

2.3 Antibodies ... 25

2.4 Solutions and buffers ... 26

2.5 Composition of gels for SDS-PAGE ... 26

2.6 Equipment ... 27

2.7 Software ... 28

3 Methods ... 29

3.1 Primary midbrain neuronal cultures ... 29
3.1.1 Experimental animals ... 29
3.1.2 Coating the coverslips and culture plates ... 29
3.1.3 Preparation of primary midbrain neurons ... 29

3.2 Transfection of PMN cultures with miRNA mimics ... 30

3.3 Measuring miRNA levels for transfection amount study ... 31
3.3.1 RNA Isolation from PMN cultures ... 31
3.3.2 RNA and DNA quantification ... 31
3.3.3 Reverse transcription ... 32
3.3.4 Quantitative real time polymerase chain reaction ... 32

3.4 Neurodegeneration models *in vitro* 33
3.4.1 Scratch lesion model 33
3.4.2 1-Methyl-4-phenylpyridinium (MPP^+) treatment 33
3.5 Immunocytochemistry 34
3.5.1 Fixation, staining and preparation for immunocytochemistry of PMN 34
3.5.2 Immunocytochemistry imaging 35
3.5.3 Evaluation of immunocytochemistry photomicrographs 35
3.6 Proteome analysis of miRNA transfected PMN 35
3.6.1 Preparation of cell lysates from PMN 35
3.6.2 Protein quantification and processing of cell lysates 36
3.6.3 LC/MS/MS on PMN protein lysates 36
3.6.4 Interpretation of SWATH-MS data and miRNA target prediction 38
3.6.5 Western blot 38
3.7 Statistical analysis 39
4 Results 40
4.1 Transfection of PMN with different doses of miRNA mimics 40
4.2 Increased levels of miR-132-3p enhanced neurite growth in dopaminergic PMN 41
4.3 Elevated levels of miR-132-3p improve regeneration of dopaminergic neurites after scratch lesion 42
4.4 Neither miR-132-3p nor miR-212-3p mimics have neuroprotective effects in MPP^+ treated dopaminergic PMN 44
4.5 miR-7b-5p and miR-129-2-3p do not alter neurite growth, neurite regeneration or survival of dopaminergic PMN 45
4.6 LC/MS/MS proteome analysis of miR-132-3p and miR-212-3p transfected PMN 47
4.7 Analysis of protein expression in miR-132-3p and miR-212-3p treated PMN by Western blot 51
5 Discussion 55
5.1 Modelling miRNA overexpression in PMN 55
5.2 Possible mechanisms of increased neurite growth in miR-132-3p mimics treated dopaminergic PMN 55
5.3 miR-132-3p induced improvement of neurite regeneration in dopaminergic PMN and possible underlying mechanisms 58
5.4 Transfection with miR-132-3p or miR-212-3p mimics cannot protect dopaminergic neurons from MPP^+ induced toxicity 59
5.5 SWATH-MS and target validation in Western blot 61
5.6 Possible mechanisms and pathways mediating the effects observed in ICC 64
5.7 miR-132-3p and miR-212-3p show different effects in neurite growth and regeneration experiments 67
5.8 Concluding remarks 70
6 Summary 71
7 Appendix 72
8 References 78

1 Introduction

The discovery of antibiotics, the increasing use of vaccination and improving neonatal care in the 20th century led to an increased life expectancy from 50 years to currently more than 80 years in developed countries. Consequently, the focus of practitioners and medical research shifted from infectious diseases to age related disorders whose incidence and prevalence increased dramatically with increasing life expectancy. This includes among others ischemic cardiovascular diseases, cancer and neurodegenerative diseases (ND) (Niccoli and Partridge 2012; Lunenfeld and Stratton 2013). Investigating ND is particularly interesting as the affected neurons are post-mitotic cells. They cannot replicate, have limited abilities to regenerate and can thus be a limiting factor of life expectancy and quality of life in ND such as Alzheimer's disease (AD) or Parkinson's disease (PD). These two most common ND are chronic progressive diseases affecting predominantly elderly people and consequently show increasing incidence and prevalence due to the demographic changes (Savica et al. 2016). The movement disorder PD is diagnosed based on clinical symptoms without objective disease specific biomarkers. It can only be treated symptomatically without possibilities to prevent disease progression. Pathophysiologically, PD is hallmarked by a loss of dopaminergic projections from the midbrain to the striatum. However, the reasons for this neuron loss are still unclear. Other regions, however, are also affected at different times during disease development.

A new field of research was opened by the discovery of various epigenetic influences determining the phenotype of cells and organisms besides their pure sequence of the deoxyribonucleotide acid (DNA) – their genome. In this context, microRNA (miRNA, RNA = ribonucleotide acid) regulating gene expression by inhibition of protein translation were described. Just as several other epigenetic mechanisms, they can be influenced by the environment and their alterations can be partially inherited. They are investigated as putative biomarkers, parts of pathomechanisms and are putative therapeutic agents or targets in PD and many other diseases (Waddington 2012; Chakraborty et al. 2017; Roser et al. 2018a).

1.1 Parkinson's disease

1.1.1 Different types of Parkinsonian syndromes

The French neurologist Jean-Martin Charcot (1825-1893) first suggested the term "Parkinson's disease" for the syndrome (a set of symptoms) James Parkinson described in "An Essay on the Shaking Palsy" in 1817. Parkinson's report characterized bradykinesia, rigidity, tremor and postural and gait impairment as the cardinal symptoms of a disease that he observed in six patients, some of which he could not even examine. Charcot later described the clinical features much more exactly, identified clinical subtypes and distinguished PD from multiple sclerosis (MS) and amyotrophic lateral sclerosis (ALS). Different diseases can clinically appear with a Parkinsonian syndrome (Goetz 2011; Mhyre et al. 2012; Jankovic 2015).

Idiopathic Parkinson's Disease is the more precise name for a Parkinsonian syndrome which is not inherited and cannot be attributed to any secondary disease-causing reasons. It is the most frequent (~ 80%) diagnosis for patients with Parkinson's syndrome (Dauer and Przedborski 2003; Mhyre et al. 2012).

Monogenic (or familial) Parkinsonian syndrome due to specific monogenetic changes and its inheritance follows Mendelian Laws. It is estimated that 5 % - 10 % of all PD cases can be explained by monogenic inheritance but 15 % - 20 % have a positive family history for PD (Gasser et al. 2011; Nuytemans et al. 2010). Familial PD often stands out with an early onset of disease. The different types of inherited PD have specific courses and treatment response depending on the responsible gene and mutation. The number of affected genes, and genetic risk factors increases constantly (Lill 2016; Zhang et al. 2018; Klein and Westenberger 2012; Coppede 2012).

Atypical Parkinsonian syndromes (aPS) are a group of ND where a Parkinsonian syndrome can also be observed. Additionally, patients suffer from subtype specific symptoms and often only poorly respond to dopamine replacing therapies. This group includes progressive supranuclear palsy (PSP), multiple system atrophy (MSA), corticobasal degeneration (CBD) and Dementia with Lewy bodies (DLB) (Mitra et al. 2003; Thenganatt and Jankovic 2014; Jankovic 2015).

In cases of **secondary Parkinsonian syndrome**, the symptoms can be attributed to a specific disease-causing reason. Drug induced Parkinsonism is the second-most-common reason for a Parkinsonian syndrome – in certain contexts also known as extrapyramidal (drug) side effects. Secondary PD may come from treatment with dopamine antagonistic drugs such as lithium, valproic acid, antipsychotics (e.g. chlorpromazine, risperidone), antiemetics (e.g. metoclopramide), certain calcium channel blockers (e.g. flunarizine) and other drugs (Shin and Chung 2012). Parkinsonism can also be induced by trauma, inflammation (e.g. AIDS, encephalopathy), metabolic disorders (e.g. Morbus Wilson, Hypoparathyroidism) or toxins like the pesticides paraquat, rotenone and others (Lee and Gilbert 2016).

Pathologically, neurodegenerative diseases can be classified according to the different protein aggregates. PD, MSA and DLB are classified as a α-synucleinopathies. Whereas α-synuclein aggregates are found as intraneuronal Lewy bodies in PD and DLB, in MSA they are described as inclusion bodies in oligodendroglia. In contrast, PSP, CBD and AD can be classified as tauopathies (Mitra et al. 2003; Halliday et al. 2011).

1.1.2 Epidemiology of Parkinson's disease

Among neurodegenerative diseases, PD is the second most common disorder after AD. The prevalence of PD in a general unselected population in industrialized countries is about 0.1 % - 0.4 %. In people older than 60 years it becomes about 1.0 % up to 3.0 % among people of 80 years and older (de Rijk et al. 2000). Incidence rates differ between 10 to more than 20 per 100,000 people per year (Tysnes and Storstein 2017; Lee and Gilbert 2016; de Rijk et al. 1995). With age as a main risk factor for PD and increasing life expectancies worldwide, prevalence and incidence of PD are also increasing (Savica et al. 2016). The median age of onset of PD symptoms was believed to be about 60 years, with a life time risk of developing the disease of 1.5 % (Lees et al. 2009). Recently published studies however described a median age of disease onset between 70.6 up to 74 years (Tysnes and Storstein 2017; Savica et al. 2016).

Different epidemiological studies have shown a significant higher prevalence and incidence in men, about 1.5 to 2.0 times higher than in women. Moreover, age at onset can be later in women and the phenotype of PD is often milder than in men. Estrogen is therefore controversially discussed as a possible neuroprotective factor. Various disease risk modifying factors were identified through epidemiological studies but many of the (exposure dependent) risk increasing factors are more linked to secondary PD. On the other hand, some of the putative protective factors are even tested for therapeutic potential. (Lee and Gilbert 2016; de Lau and Breteler 2006).

1.1.3 Pathophysiology and pathogenesis of Parkinson's disease

1.1.3.1 Pathophysiology of Parkinson's disease

When James Parkinson gave his famous description for the syndrome which was later named after him, he suspected the disease's focus to be in the central nervous system (CNS) most likely in the spinal cord or the *medulla oblongata* (part of the brainstem). He could not imagine other CNS parts to be the focus of the disease as he did not observe any sense or intellectual impairments (Parkinson 2002). It took until the beginning of the 20th century until a degeneration of dopaminergic neurons in the *substantia nigra pars compacta* (SNpc) of the mesencephalon was described in patients with Parkinsonian syndrome (Goedert et al. 2013; Lingor et al. 2017). The loss of dopaminergic projections from the SNpc to the striatum leads to a reduced disinhibition of the motoric thalamus and subsequently to a general inhibition of movement. The more nigrostriatal projections are lost, the stronger the motor inhibition and disease symptoms become (Bernheimer et al. 1973; Bertler and Rosengren 1959, 1966).

1.1.3.2 Pathogenesis of Parkinson's disease

The dysfunction in the motoric coordinating circuit of striatum, substantia nigra and thalamus plausibly explain the characteristic motor symptoms observed in PD. However, the reasons for the loss of the nigrostriatal projections are not yet elucidated. Mitochondrial dysfunction, oxidative stress, protein mishandling and aggregation as well as various environmental factors are discussed as possible parts of the pathogenesis of PD. Important knowledge on PD pathogenesis is derived from mutations observed in familial PD. Even before the loss of dopaminergic neurons was described as a pivotal pathophysiological mechanism, the *substantia nigra* was known as the locus of PD. In 1912, Friedrich Heinrich Lewy discovered inclusion bodies in various brain parts of PD patients which were later named Lewy bodies. Decades later, a rare type of autosomal dominantly inherited PD was attributed to mutations in the α-synuclein gene (*SNCA*). Shortly thereafter, Spillantini and colleagues demonstrated that aggregated α-synuclein is a major component of Lewy bodies also in non-familial PD (Goedert et al. 2013; Polymeropoulos et al. 1997; Spillantini et al. 1997). The distribution of α-synuclein correlates to the clinical disease stage. In early stages, only the brainstem and the anterior olfactory nucleus are affected – in later stages, other brain areas become affected in a specific order (Braak et al. 2003).

The disease stage-dependent distribution of α-synuclein led to two hypotheses. First, α-synuclein spreads through the brain in a prion-like manner. Thus, the disease phenotype should be modeled by α-synuclein inoculation. Cell to cell transmission of α-synuclein was already observed in different cell culture models (Angot et al. 2010; Luk et al. 2012). Even in fetal human midbrain neurons transplanted into PD patients' midbrains, α-synuclein was detected already four years after transplantation (Chu and Kordower 2010). In contrast to true prion diseases like scrapie or Creutzfeldt Jakob Disease (CJD), an infectivity of misfolded α-synuclein and a subsequent induction of α-synuclein aggregation, has not yet been observed neither in human nor in animal models (Angot et al. 2010).

The second hypothesis deals with the fact that the spread of α-synuclein seems to have starting points – one in the anterior olfactory nucleus and one in the brainstem close to the dorsal nucleus of the vagal nerve. Compared to controls, PD patients had more aggregates of α-synuclein in the enteral plexus of Auerbach and Meissner (Wakabayashi et al. 1988). Furthermore, a Danish cohort study showed a tendency to a reduced risk to develop PD for patients who underwent truncal vagotomy (Svensson et al. 2015) – a suspicion that could not be confirmed in a similar Swedish cohort (Liu et al. 2017). However, the affection of the vagal system correlates well with constipation, hypotension and sleep disorders observed in PD patients. Besides, alterations in the gut microbiome are described and even efforts to use it as diagnostic biomarker were made (Scheperjans et al. 2015). Both hypotheses indicate that PD might be triggered by an exogenous pathogen entering through the enteral system and the nose – the dual hit hypothesis (Hawkes et al. 2007).

It still must be investigated whether or how exactly α-synuclein harms selectively dopaminergic neurons, how it is possibly transmitted between cells and how its aggregation is induced. Whereas some studies did not observe α-synuclein-induced degeneration or cell death (Tompkins and Hill 1997; Parkkinen et al. 2011), most reports described an α-synuclein-induced impairment of synaptic functions, cytoskeletal remodeling, mitochondria or protein degradation subsequently leading to neurodegeneration. Besides, overexpression of α-synuclein is frequently used in animal models of PD (Stefanis 2012). A malfunction of the protein-degrading ubiquitin proteasome system (UPS) is discussed to be involved in α-synuclein aggregation as mutations in the UPS related *PARKIN* gene were observed in familial PD. Still, it was also demonstrated that α-synuclein can aggregate independently of the UPS (Moore et al. 2003; Kitada et al. 1998; Lim 2007; Giasson and Lee 2003; Sampathu et al. 2003). Besides, the discovery of *GBA1* mutations – a gene encoding for the lysosomal enzyme glucocerebrosidase – as a genetic risk factor for developing PD, has driven the attention to lysosomes as a part of PD pathogenesis. Also, the common mutations in *LRRK2* or *DJ-1* in familial PD and various other genetic risk factors could be linked to failures in lysosomal pathways. For instance, increased levels of oxidized dopamine were reported to lead to an acquired reduction of glucocerebrosidase activity and mitochondrial failure in dopaminergic neurons from induced pluripotent stem cells from homozygous *DJ-1* mutated PD patients. The lysosomal dysfunction is also suspected to be involved in the accumulation of α-synuclein in PD patients' brains (Kilpatrick 2016; Burbulla et al. 2017).

Apart from that, most mutated genes in familial PD (e.g. *PINK1, PARKIN, LRRK2, SNCA*) can be linked to increased vulnerability and instability of mitochondria and impaired degradation (mitophagy). Besides, mitochondrial dysfunction was also observed in sporadic PD. Moreover, several cases of secondary Parkinsonism in patients with intravenous drug abuse could be attributed to toxins harming mitochondria in dopaminergic neurons. (Davis et al. 1979; Langston et al. 1983; Park et al. 2018). The opioid drugs were contaminated with 1-Methyl-4-phenyl-1,2,3,6-tetrahydropyridine (MPTP) which was later described to be oxidized by astrocytes' monoaminoxidase type B (MAO-B) to 1-methyl-4-phenylpyridinium (MPP^+). Through dopamine transporters, MPP^+ specifically enters dopaminergic neurons and inhibits the mitochondrial complex I, which increases levels of *reactive oxygen species* (ROS) and impairs the cells' energy supply. Today, complex I inhibitors such as MPP^+ or 6-hydroxydopamine are frequently used in various models of PD (Corsini et al. 1987; Kopin 1992; Gerlach et al. 1991; Dauer and Przedborski 2003). Mutations in mitochondrial complex I could be identified as a risk factor for developing PD but also dementia (Yan et al. 2013). Furthermore, complex I inhibition was observed throughout the entire brain of sporadic PD patients but the substantia nigra was the only analyzed brain part where it correlated with DNA damage (Schapira et al. 1990; Mann et al. 1994; Janetzky et al. 1994). Interestingly, α-synuclein aggregation was decreased in complex I deficient neurons (Flønes et al. 2018; Dölle et al. 2016).

Possible reasons for the particular vulnerability of dopaminergic neurons to an impaired mitochondrial and complex I function might be the constant production of ROS through dopamine metabolism (Miyazaki and Asanuma 2008; Hastings 2009). On the other hand, dopamine depletion neither protects from MPTP toxicity (Hasbani et al. 2005) nor does dopamine replacing therapy accelerate the progression of PD (Fahn 2005). Thus, dopamine metabolism is possibly not the major or at least not the only reason for the vulnerability of dopaminergic neurons. However, α-synuclein was reported to induce mitochondrial fragmentation both in wild type and in different mutants by destabilizing the mitochondrial membrane (Ryan et al. 2015; Park et al. 2018). Furthermore, a special type of voltage gated calcium channels in SNpc dopaminergic neurons with increased calcium influx was described to increases oxidative stress and energy consumption. Interestingly, dihydropyridine calcium channel blockers were reported to lower the risk of developing PD. Although, PD patients tend to have low blood pressure, which makes the drugs – normally used to treat hypertension – less appropriate for treatment of PD. Clinical trials could however not demonstrate a therapeutic effect of dihydropyridine (Kilpatrick 2016).

Like in various other neurodegenerative diseases an accumulation of iron is observed in PD patients' brains, which however, also increases physiologically with age. Nevertheless, iron can induce translation of α-synuclein and probably enhances its aggregation (Lingor et al. 2017). Moreover, iron is a co-factor of several redox enzymes and its homeostasis is important to control ROS as high iron levels can induce oxidative stress and increased iron levels can also be involved in mitochondrial damage (Zecca et al. 2004; Park et al. 2018). Furthermore, upregulation of inflammatory markers can be observed in PD patients and inflammation (including an activation of microglia and astrocytes) is probably contributing to the disease's progression. Still, inflammation or immune response are most likely not the main disease-causing mechanisms (Tufekci et al. 2012).

At the time the first motor symptoms appear, already 60 - 80 % of the dopaminergic neurons in the SNpc have died and even more nigrostriatal projections have been lost – an observation which led to the "dying back hypothesis" of a degeneration starting in the distal axon (Burke and O'Malley 2013; Tagliaferro and Burke 2016; Dauer and Przedborski 2003). Burke and O'Malley proposed that the degeneration of nigrostriatal axons is contributing more to the development of PD symptoms than the neuronal loss in the SN. Neurites are especially vulnerable to ROS or impaired energy supply and α-synuclein was demonstrated to impair cytoskeletal remodeling. Thus, they assumed that better understanding of axon growth, their degeneration and regeneration could lead to new therapeutic and possibly disease modifying therapies for PD.

1.1.4 Symptoms and diagnostics of Parkinson's disease

1.1.4.1 Clinical symptoms of Parkinson's disease

James Parkinson described the originally *Paralysis agitans* (Shaking Palsy) called disease as an "involuntary tremulous motion, with lessened muscular power, in parts not in action [..]; with a propensity to bend the trunk forwards" (Parkinson 2002). The rest tremor and the impaired gait were the most obvious symptoms. Four cardinal symptoms were identified for what is now known as Parkinson's syndrome: bradykinesia, rest tremor, rigidity and postural and gait impairment. Beside these motor symptoms also non-motor symptoms were described which were not part of Parkinson's original description (Massano and Bhatia 2012; Clarke 2007).

Bradykinesia describes the reduced pace of the patients in all their actions and their disability to rapidly alternate movements (*dysdiadochokinesia*). Hypomimia ("Poker face", reduced mimic), hypophonia (unclear, soft voice) and micrographia (progressively smaller handwriting towards the end of a line) also belong to the summarizing term bradykinesia. The predominantly rhythmic 4-6 Hz **rest tremor** mostly affects relaxed body parts and vanishes with active movement (Massano and Bhatia 2012). Although in public perception, tremor is the most typical symptom of PD only 48 % of male and 67 % of female patients show it. The Parkinsonian rest tremor must not be confused with the essential tremor which has a prevalence between 0.4 % and 3.9 % in a general population (Zesiewicz and Kuo 2015). The **rigidity** observed in PD is also described as cogwheel rigidity. In difference to spastic palsy the Parkinsonian rigidity is felt throughout the entire movement and does not increase (Massano and Bhatia 2012). The "propensity to bend the trunk forwards" observed by Parkinson is today described as **postural and gait impairment.** Patients turn around in multiple small steps and fall easily (Jankovic 2015).

Besides these relatively obvious motor symptoms, PD patients also suffer from several neuropsychiatric (e.g. dementia, depression, psychosis, apathy), vegetative (e.g. hyposmia, dysphagia, constipation, sexual dysfunction, orthostatic hypotension) and sleep disorders (especially rapid eye movement sleep disorders, RBD) as well as pain, fatigue and sensory dysfunction. These complaints are important to asses as they can heavily impair the quality of life of patients and should also be treated (Massano and Bhatia 2012; Clarke 2007). Moreover, these complaints can occur in early stages of the disease even before the onset of motor symptoms and are therefore important to monitor when dealing with elderly and other risk patients to diagnose PD early (Miller and O'Callaghan 2015; Oertel and Schulz 2016).

The disease progresses very differently and life expectancy, quality of life or degree of disability differ a lot between patients. A better sub-classification of PD is needed for more precise prognosis, specific treatment and significant studies. Clinically, three subtypes are differentiated according to the leading clinical symptom: an akinetic rigid type, a tremor dominant type and an equivalent type. More precise classification systems also include age at onset, a larger set of symptoms or biomarkers for differentiation (Thenganatt and Jankovic 2014; Fereshtehnejad et al. 2015; Eggers et al. 2012). Besides the tremor-dominant phenotype, also a benign tremulous PD is described with poor levodopa (L-Dopa) response and only mild progression of other PD symptoms. It is therefore discussed to possibly be a unique disease (Deeb et al. 2016; Josephs et al. 2006).

Moreover, histological differences between clinical PD subtypes were reported. Patients with non-tremor dominant PD were described to have significantly more amyloid-β-plaques and Lewy bodies in the cortex compared to tremor dominant or early onset PD subtypes (Halliday et al. 2011; Selikhova et al. 2009).

1.1.4.2 Establishing the diagnosis of idiopathic Parkinson's disease

The diagnosis of PD follows the criteria of the Movement Disorder Society and starts with the identification of a Parkinsonian syndrome consisting of the indispensable bradykinesia and at least one out of rest tremor or rigidity. Subsequently, absolute exclusion criteria e.g. dealing with reasons of secondary Parkinsonism and aPS related symptoms are ruled out. Secondly, at least two supportive criteria such as olfactory loss or improvement after dopaminergic therapy shall be identified. Third, red flags such as bilateral symmetric symptoms, unusual rapid or slow progression are excluded for the diagnosis of *clinically established PD*. *Clinically probable PD* can be diagnosed if not more than two red flags are each counterbalanced by supportive criteria (Postuma et al. 2015a).

Thus, the diagnosis relies on the clinical examination and the expertise of the neurologist but additional examinations in blood or cerebrospinal fluid (CSF) and general neuroimaging techniques can help to exclude other rare causes of the observed symptoms. A hyper-echogenic substantia nigra in transcranial sonography may support the diagnosis of PD but cannot differentiate from atypical Parkinsonism. Single photon emission computed tomography (SPECT) of the of presynaptic dopamine transporters (so-called DaTSCAN) can help to support the diagnosis especially by differentiating between an essential tremor and Parkinson's disease. Costly but helpful even in the difficult differentiation of PD to some aPS, is the Positron-emission tomography with ^{18}fluoro-dopa, ^{18}fluoro-deoxy-glucose (^{18}FDG) or ^{18}C-raclopride (Tolosa et al. 2006; Miller and O'Callaghan 2015).

The course of the disease can clinically be documented with the Hoehn and Yahr scale or the Unified Parkinson's Disease Rating Scale (UPDRS). The neuropathological postmortem diagnosis of PD is defined by neuronal loss in the SNpc and Lewy body pathology which can be grouped by Braak stages (Dickson et al. 2009).

Only 75 % to 95 % of the experts' PD diagnosis are confirmed on autopsy. The accuracy of PD diagnosis considerably depends on disease duration and the expert's experience. Not recognizing warning signals for atypical Parkinsonism is one of the main diagnostic errors.

Thus, the diagnosis of PD hast to be questioned regularly (Postuma et al. 2015a; Postuma et al. 2018). To diagnose PD earlier, proofed by objective parameters and to better differentiate PD and aPS, neurologist strive for PD biomarkers. In this context, different metabolites, proteins, elements and also miRNAs are investigated in various material such as blood, CSF, urine and tear fluid (Stoicea et al. 2016; Miller and O'Callaghan 2015). Even skin biopsies are considered for PD diagnosis as phosphorylated-α-synuclein deposits could be found in skin nerves of 80 % to 100 % of the examined PD patients but not in healthy controls. Interestingly, some patients with RBD – an early symptom of PD – were also positive for phosphorylated-α-synuclein (Doppler et al. 2017; Donadio et al. 2014; Postuma et al. 2015b).

1.1.5 Treatment of Parkinson's disease

So far, there is still no disease-modifying therapy available for PD. Instead, symptoms are treated by dopamine replacement since the degeneration of nigrostriatal dopaminergic projections is the best-understood part in PD pathophysiology. Patients below the age of 70 are often first treated with a non-ergotamine dopamine agonist such as pramipexol, ropinirole or rotigotine. All patients with PD, however, benefit of a treatment with the precursor substance levodopa (L-Dopa, 3,4-hydroxyphenylalanin). In contrast to dopamine, it crosses the blood-brain barrier and gets then decarboxylated to dopamine. To prevent peripheral side effects, L-Dopa is always combined with a peripheral decarboxylase inhibitor like benserazide or carbidopa (Bentley and Sharma 2012; Oertel and Schulz 2016). Drugs are usually applied orally. For the dopamine agonists, also subcutaneous (apomorphine) or transdermal (rotigotine) applications are available. L-Dopa is also available as slow release preparation or can be applied as intrajejunal infusion (Duodopa pump) for patients with severe motor fluctuations (Oertel and Schulz 2016; Olanow et al. 2014). When fluctuations of therapeutic response occur, therapy with L-Dopa or dopamine agonists can be supported by inhibiting dopamine degradation using catechol-O-methyl transferase (COMT)-inhibitors (entacapone, opicapone, tolcapone) or MAO-B inhibitors (rasagiline, safinamide, selegiline) (Oertel and Schulz 2016). Besides, some patients can be helped with deep brain stimulation (DBS) of the *subthalamic nucleus, globus pallidus pars interna* or the *ventral intermediate nucleus* which physiologically inhibit the motoric thalamus. The electric stimulus of the DBS inhibits these centers leading to a disinhibition of the motoric thalamus and thereby taking over the effects physiologically elicited by dopaminergic nigrostriatal projections. Especially young patients with L-Dopa induced motor fluctuations or non-levodopa-responsive tremor can profit from DBS (Moldovan et al. 2015; Oertel and Schulz 2016; Herrington et al. 2016).

In addition to pharmacological treatment, physical therapy, occupational therapy, speech therapy as well as cognitive behavioral therapy are important to maintain patients' self-sustainment and social participation (Gage and Storey 2004; Keus et al. 2007).

Many different strategies have been considered to provide a disease-modifying treatment to PD patients. Of course, this research could also benefit enormously from advances in biomarker research, better sub-classification of PD types and earlier diagnosis of the disease. Future treatment strategies focus on certain parts of the pathogeneses of PD or putative protective factors identified in epidemiological studies. It was observed that PD appears less frequent in smokers than in non-smokers and even leads to altered MAO-B activity in smokers. However, a clinical trial using nicotine as therapy did not slow down disease progression and even worsens symptoms compared to placebo control (Oertel et al. 2018). The apparent protective effect of smoking can be explained by a lower life expectancy of smokers and less addiction potential due to reduced dopamine levels in PD, which makes it easier for PD patients to quit smoking (Ritz et al. 2014; Lee and Gilbert 2016; de Lau and Breteler 2006). Other factors which are suggested to reduce the risk of developing PD are nonsteroidal anti-inflammatory drugs and statins which also have anti-inflammatory properties. As drinking coffee is suspected to be a protective factor against developing PD, caffeine was also tested for PD treatment but could not improve patients' motor symptoms in a randomized placebo-controlled trial (Postuma et al. 2017). Moreover, high levels of urate are suspected to reduce the risk of developing PD. Different safety trials with the urate precursor inosine have already shown the safety of the drug and its ability to raise serum and CSF levels of urate. Treatment effects of inosine in PD are currently evaluated in clinical trials (Schwarzschild et al. 2014; Iwaki et al. 2017; Oertel and Schulz 2016). In the context of possible risk and protective factors, it is important to underline, that most of these factors were identified retrospectively using questionnaires which are susceptible to recall bias.

Since a prion like behavior of α-synuclein is discussed, clinical trials try to limit extracellular α-synuclein levels to stop further spread through the brain and cell death. Active and passive immunotherapies are undergoing clinical phase I or II trials and have not reported any serious side effects so far (Oertel and Schulz 2016). Moreover, iron – which is suspected to support intracellular α-synuclein aggregation – is also investigated as a putative treatment target. In preclinical studies using the A53T mouse model of PD, the iron chelator deferiprone and the selective inhibitor of iron-α-synuclein-interaction clioquinol improved behavioral deficits (Carboni et al. 2017; Finkelstein et al. 2016). Deferiprone is even tested in a large scale clinical trial in patients in early stages of PD (Martin-Bastida et al. 2017).

Regarding oxidative stress and mitochondrial dysfunction as a possible part of PD pathogenesis, a phase III trial with coenzyme Q10 – a mitochondrial enhancer and antioxidant – could not show any benefit for the patients – possibly since the general collective of PD patients is still too heterogenous (Beal et al. 2014; Oertel and Schulz 2016).

Transplantation of human embryonic dopaminergic neurons to patients with severe PD only led to an improvement in patients below the age of 60 years (Freed et al. 2001). In another similar study, no benefit for the patient was observed but more "off" dyskinesia in treated patients (Olanow et al. 2003). Further pharmacological and interventional treatment trials as well as basic research are required to identify biomarkers and elucidate pathogenesis of PD to provide a better symptom controlling or even disease modifying treatment to PD patients.

1.2 Epigenetics

The DNA sequence is the building plan of cells and organisms. However, only ~2 % of the DNA fulfill this original building plan hypothesis and encode for proteins (Venter et al. 2001; Alexander et al. 2010). Thus, the pure DNA sequence is probably not everything what determines the phenotype of an organism. Long before DNA sequences were revealed, Conrad Waddington supposed in 1942 that "between genotype and phenotype […] lies a whole complex of developmental processes" which he called the "epigenotype" (Waddington 2012).

Epigenetic mechanisms can modify gene expression in different stages. DNA methylation or histone modifications alter the transcription of RNA from the DNA template strands by regulating the DNA strands' accessibility for transcription enzymes or factors. This can be an important part of cell differentiation but can also be transmitted to following cell or organism generations via enzymes copying this epigenetic code during meiosis or mitosis (Gibney and Nolan 2010; Riggs and Porter 1996; Bird 2007). Besides, gene expression can be modified on a post-transcriptional level during processing of the precursor messenger RNA (pre-mRNA) or finally upon translation of the messenger RNA (mRNA). During post-transcriptional processing, most pre-mRNA transcripts are alternatively spliced, introns are removed and (some of) the remaining exons are rearranged. Additionally, high specific base exchanges like A-to-I editing or C-to-U-editing increases the variability in protein synthesis. In average, 6.3 alternatively spliced transcripts come from one gene locus but one mature mRNA only encodes for one protein (ENCODE Project Consortium 2012; Brennicke et al. 1999).

Other RNA transcripts do not encode for protein but control mRNA translation. In 2006, Andrew Fire and Craig C. Mello were awarded the Nobel Prize for Medicine and Physiology for their description of genetic interference by double stranded RNA (dsRNA). A foundation-stone for their research was laid by Lee and colleagues in 1993 who described an RNA transcript later called **microRNA** (miRNA, ~21 to 25 nucleotides) from a non-coding gene which specifically regulated the translation of a mRNA by antisense RNA-RNA interaction (Fire et al. 1998; Lee et al. 1993). Moreover, **small interfering RNA** (siRNA, ~21 to 25 nucleotides) processed by cleavage from exogenous (e.g. viral) or endogenous RNA duplexes were described as well as the single stranded **Piwi-interacting RNA** (piRNA, ~24-29 nucleotides long). All these three interfering RNAs need to interact with Argonaut proteins to bind to their targets. Alterations in their expression regulate gene expression, can be acquired and inherited (Siomi and Siomi 2009; Houwing et al. 2007; Heard and Martienssen 2014; Benito et al. 2018; Smythies et al. 2014).

Inheritance of these epigenetic modifications could possibly mean that cells and organisms take over the adaptation of their ancestors – one of the key ideas of Jean-Baptiste Lamarck's theory of evolution (1744-1829). Environment induced epigenetic modifications could thus influence gene expression, cognitive abilities, disease risks and even fears (Dias and Ressler 2013; Fischer 2014).

1.3 miRNA in epigenetic regulation

miRNAs are a group of non-coding RNA usually between 21 to 25 nucleotides long. They are transcribed from DNA mostly by RNA polymerase (RNA Pol) II or III which leads to a stem-loop structure – the primary miRNA (pri-miRNA). Many pri-miRNAs are capped at their 5' end and are polyadenylated at the 3' end just as mRNA. The RNAse III Drosha (also called microprocessor complex) together with the dsRNA binding protein DGCR8 then cleaves the pri-miRNA which results in an about 65-70 nucleotides long precursor miRNA (pre-miRNA). In some cases, a cluster of two to seven pre-miRNA is processed from one common pri-miRNA. The transport protein Exportin-5 (XPO5) in complex with Ran-GTP then recognizes the pre-miRNA by its hairpin structure and its 3' overhang and transports only correctly processed pre-miRNA into the cytoplasm. In the cytoplasm, the evolutionary conserved RNAse III Dicer processes the pre-miRNA into a ~21 to 25 nucleotides long duplex RNA with two nucleotides overhang on the 3' end. Afterwards, the double stranded mature miRNA becomes separated, possibly by miRNA specific enzymes.

The miRNA strand which has its 5' end at the site of the thermodynamically less stable base pair is selected as the guide strand whereas the passenger strand usually is degraded. Finally, the selected guide strand is loaded into the RNA induced silencing complex (RISC). It always contains an Argonaute 1 or (more often) Argonaute 2 protein (Ago 1 or 2) and more miRNA specific proteins. Dicer and dsRNA unwinding enzymes are suspected to assist in this process. The RISC binds especially to the mRNA's 3' untranslated region by more or less perfect base pairing of the loaded miRNA to the target mRNA. Base pairing is suspected to depend especially on the seed sequence between the 2nd and 8th nucleotide of the miRNA's 5' side. However, besides complementary base pairing miRNA targeting probably also depends on factors such as miRNA confirmation or accessibility of the target. After pairing to its target, RISC can cleave mRNA, inhibit mRNA translation or promote mRNA degradation. The exact effect probably differs between species, different miRNA and could (among others) depend on the grade of base complementarity (Winter et al. 2009; Siomi and Siomi 2009; Ameres and Zamore 2013; Didiano and Hobert 2006; Wang 2014).

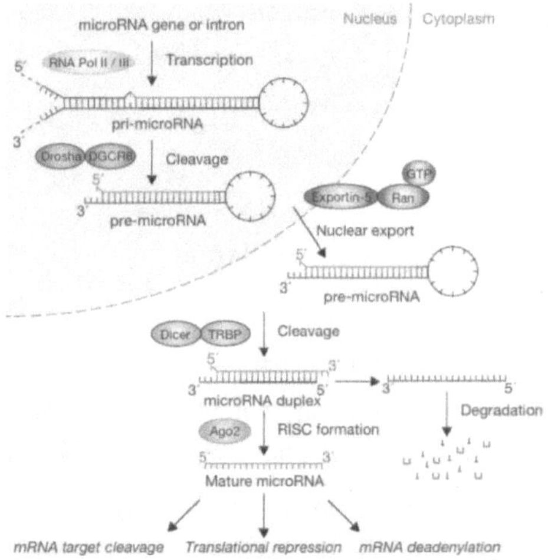

Figure 1 Canonical pathway of miRNA biogenesis

The pri-miRNA is transcribed by RNA polymerase II or III, cleaved to a shorter pre-miRNA by Drosha and exported to the cytoplasm via Exportin-5. In the cytoplasm it is cleaved by Dicer, one miRNA strand is selected (in this case the red labeled 5'-3' strand) and is loaded into RISC whereas the other strand is degraded. RISC and its loaded miRNA target an mRNA by complementary base pairing and thereby regulate mRNA translation. With kind permission of Springer Nature, Winter et al. 2009.

Besides this canonical pathway other Drosha and/or Dicer independent pathways are described. Intron derived (intragenic) miRNAs can be processed independently of Drosha if the initial splicing results in a hairpin RNA with a size like a pre-miRNA. Regarding transcription, intragenic miRNAs can both be transcribed and processed with the respective gene but also independently controlled by specific promoters (Winter et al. 2009; Wang et al. 2013b).

The biogenesis of miRNAs can be regulated at different levels. First, just as gene expression, miRNA biogenesis can be regulated by DNA methylation (many miRNAs are located in CpG islands) and post-transcriptional modifications of histones. Among others, this alters the DNA's accessibility for a second regulatory mechanism of gene expression – the binding of transcription factors to specific promotors. For many miRNAs specific transcription factors are described (Wang et al. 2013b). Interestingly, even miRNA which were transcribed as a cluster, can be regulated independently (Song and Wang 2008; Magill et al. 2010). Third, – just as mRNAs – miRNA can be modified post-transcriptionally, among others by deamination of adenosine to inosine (A-to-I-editing). Moreover, several modifications or cofactors of miRNA processing enzymes are described to alter the biogenesis of specific miRNA (Winter et al. 2009; Wang et al. 2013b).

1.4 The miRNA cluster 132/212

1.4.1 Regulation and effects of miR-132/212

Four miRNA strands are transcribed from the miR-132/212 locus in one common pri-miRNA. In humans they are transcribed from an intergenic region on chromosome 17 p13.3. However, in mice and rats they are transcribed from introns (intragenic regions). Post-transcriptional editing or processing besides the canonical pathway of miRNA biogenesis is described for the miR-132/212 in different species. The mature miR-132-3p and miR-212-3p share a common seed sequence (5'-AACAGUC-3') and differ in only five nucleotides. Similarity of the sequence and the localization in a common gene locus probably due to evolutionary gene duplication. Moreover, both miRNA sequences are highly conserved through vertebrates suggesting an essential physiological role (Wanet et al. 2012; Vo et al. 2005).

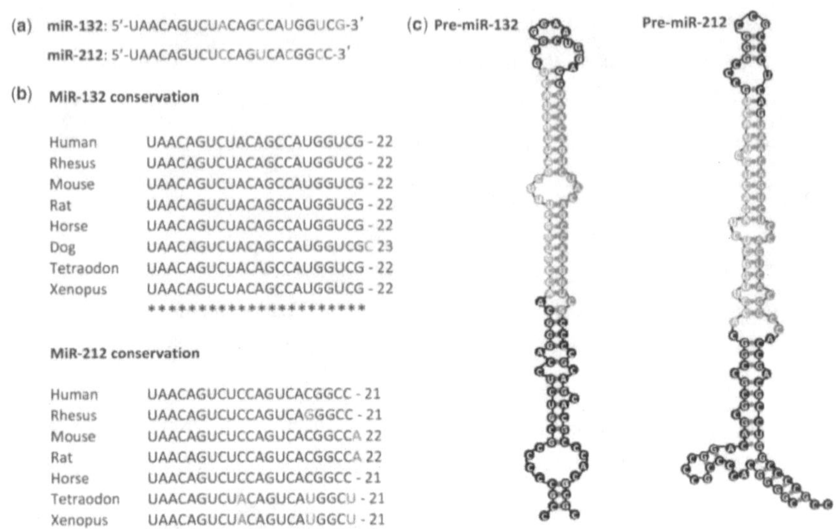

Figure 2 Structure and sequence of mature and precursor strands from the miR-132/212 cluster and its evolutionary conservation through different vertebrates

(A) The mature miRNA strands miR-132-3p and miR-212-3p share a similar sequence. Differences between the two miRNAs are highlighted in red. (B) Both mature strands are highly conserved in different vertebrates. Differences from the human sequence are highlighted in red. (C) Predicted stem-loop structure and sequence of human pre-miR-132 and pre-miR-212. The mature -3p strands are colored in red, the -5p counter strands in grey, predicted hydrogen bounds in blue. Modified from Wanet et al. 2012 under the Creative Common Attribution Non-Commercial License.

Transcription of the cluster can be induced by the cAMP-response element binding protein (CREB) and the brain-derived neurotrophic factor (BDNF) which are both involved in neuronal maturation, differentiation and plasticity. Whereas CREB has several conserved binding sites around the miR-132/212 locus, BDNF can induce its transcription indirectly via several different pathways. Some of these pathways finally regulate transcription via the regulation of CREB but also CREB independent pathways e.g. via ERK1/2 are discussed. (Vo et al. 2005; Remenyi et al. 2010). CREB can be a downstream target of BDNF effects but BDNF transcription is also directly controlled by CREB. This homeostatic control of two miR-132/212 regulating factors becomes more complicated when including the methyl-CpG-binding protein 2 (MECP2) which is a validated target of both miRNAs.

On one hand, MECP2 controls the expression of BDNF, CREB and miR-132/212. On the other hand, it is itself a target of miR-132/212 and CREB. These complex mechanisms and counter regulations probably ensures a homeostasis of all involved factors which are all crucial during maturation and neuron development (Klein et al. 2007; Feng and Nestler 2010).

Moreover, the repressor element-1 silencing transcription factor / neuron-restrictive silencing factor (REST/NRSF) has a conserved binding site to suppress miR-132/212 transcription. REST normally suppresses the expression of neuronal proteins in non-neuronal cells, but it is also present in neurons. During neuronal maturation it is proteolyzed and miR-132/212 can be transcribed (Westbrook et al. 2008; Wanet et al. 2012; Zocchi and Sassone-Corsi 2012). Interestingly, miR-132-3p was demonstrated to be the mainly expressed miRNA from this cluster in primary hippocampal cultures and the dentate gyrus of young adult mice (Magill et al. 2010).

As an epigenetic regulator of gene expression, miRNAs can adapt to the environment and miRNAs alterations can even be transmitted to the directly following generation. This was demonstrated specifically for the miR-132/212 cluster. Physical exercise and cognitive training (environmental enrichment) is known to improve performance in cognitive tasks (Fischer 2016). Mice in enriched environment developed increased levels of miR-132/212 in hippocampal and sperm specimens. The increased miRNA levels were transmitted to the following generation via the male sperm. Although the offspring mice lived in a standard environment, they still performed better in cognitive tasks compared to offspring from standard environment fathers (Benito et al. 2018).

Protein regulation by miRNAs affects a high number of targets and even more downstream targets. As the sequence of the organism specific miRNAs and its target mRNAs is known, algorithms can predict mRNAs targeted by a respected miRNA by complementary base pairing and other criteria. Sets of proteins are clustered in pathways according to the Kyoto Encyclopedia of Genes and Genomes (KEGG). An analysis of the predicted targets of the miR-132/212 seed sequence reveals various significantly affected KEGG pathways involved in the regulation of cell growth and cell cycle (Table 1). A respective table of KEGG pathways of predicted miR-132/212 targets in mice can be found in Table A1.

Table 1 The 15 most significantly affected KEGG pathways in humans according to seed-sequence-based target prediction of miR-132/212 targets by targetscan.org

KEGG pathway Term		**p-Value**
hsa04350	TGF-beta signaling pathway	3.8E-7
hsa04360	Axon guidance	6.06E-6
hsa05200	Pathways in cancer	9.0E-6
hsa04550	Signaling pathways regulating pluripotency of stem cells	8.2E-5
hsa05213	Endometrial cancer	1.7E-4
hsa04068	FoxO signaling pathway	2.4E-4
hsa04010	MAPK signaling pathway	6.7E-4
hsa04728	Dopaminergic synapse	6.8E-4
hsa05215	Prostate cancer	8.8E-4
hsa04663	B cell receptor signaling pathway	9.6E-4
hsa04022	cGMP-PKG signaling pathway	9.7E-4
hsa04917	Prolactin signaling pathway	1.1E-3
hsa05202	Transcriptional misregulation in cancer	1.5E-3
hsa04151	PI3K-Akt signaling pathway	2.3E-3
hsa04510	Focal adhesion	3.0E-2

The mature miR-132-3p strand is the best investigated strand from the miR-132/212 cluster – probably because miR-212 was discovered much later. The affected KEGG pathways of miR-132/212 include among others *Axon guidance* and *Pi3K-Akt signaling pathway* which fits well to numerous studies reporting augmented neurite outgrowth and spine density in various models with increased levels of miR-132-3p (Vo et al. 2005; Pathania et al. 2012; Magill et al. 2010; Impey et al. 2010; Hansen et al. 2010; Wayman et al. 2008). It was also reported that mild elevations of miR-132-3p levels improve performance in cognitive animal tests whereas knockout of the miR-132/212 locus worsens learning and spatial memory. In this context, the observation was explained by the miRNAs' ability to regulate neuronal plasticity and long term potentiation – possibly via their target MECP2 (Hansen et al. 2016; Hansen et al. 2013; Benito et al. 2018; Hernandez-Rapp et al. 2015; Aten et al. 2016). Moreover, a small RNA sequencing comparing primary midbrain neuronal (PMN) cultures between the first and fifth *day in vitro* (DIV) identified a massive increase in miR-132-3p and miR-212-3p expression at the later time point suggesting an essential role of these miRNAs in neuronal maturation (Roser 2016; Roser et al. 2018b). These observations suggested a further investigation of the miRNA cluster in disease contexts as growth and maturation-associated mechanisms are also suspected to be involved in regeneration.

1.4.2 miR-132/212 in disease and as therapeutic target

Pathways involved in growth or maturation – such as many of the KEGG pathways in Table 1 – are frequently also involved in cancer. One of the major suppressors of miR-132/212 transcription, REST, was observed to be downregulated in different types of cancer (Westbrook et al. 2008). Thus, alterations of miR-132/212 were described among others in pancreatic, gastric or lung cancer. Interestingly, the direction of miRNA regulation differed between studies. Although, some studies could demonstrate cancer suppressing effects of increased miR-132/212 levels, it cannot be said for sure whether the miRNA alteration is causal for cancer development, a reaction to or a consequence of it (Zhang et al. 2011; Park et al. 2011; Luo et al. 2014; Wada et al. 2010; Wanet et al. 2012).

Besides, the miR-132/212 is intensively investigated in cardiovascular diseases. As miR-132/212 targets the pro-autophagic transcription factor FOXO3, increased miR-132/212 levels are associated with the development of cardiac hypertrophy. Inhibition of miR-132-3p with antagomir (specific synthetic oligonucleotides against miRNA) could prevent cardiac hypertrophy and heart failure in mice (Ucar et al. 2012; Thum et al. 2013).

To diagnose diseases early and to estimate patients' prognosis, miRNA from different body fluids were also investigated as putative biomarkers in various diseases. For instance, the low serum levels of miR-132 and miR-212 correlate with poor survival in patients with hepatocellular carcinoma (Wang et al. 2018a) but in patients with acute myeloid leukemia high miR-212 expression is associated with a prolonged survival (Sun et al. 2013).

Furthermore, miRNAs were investigated as putative biomarkers for PD as the diagnosis is still mainly based on clinical criteria and differential diagnosis to aPS is challenging. Different body fluids such as saliva, CSF, blood and different fractions of it (CSF exosomes, whole blood, serum, blood cells) were investigated. Among the repeatedly reported miRNAs are miR-1-3p, miR-19b-3p, miR-29a-3p, miR-29c-3p, miR-214-3p, miR-221-3p. The majority of them were downregulated in PD (Roser et al. 2018a). Single miRNA could differentiate PD from healthy controls with an area under the curve (AUC) between 0.92 for miR-1-3p (downregulated) to 0.97 for miR-409-3 (upregulated) under the receiver operating characteristic (ROC) curve. Combined measurement of miR-153 and miR-409-3p in exosomes from CSF even led to an AUC of 0.99 (Gui et al. 2015). For miR-132/212 biomarker reports are contradictory. Some reports could not even detect miR-132-3p in their CSF samples (Marques et al. 2017). One study reported an upregulation of miR-132-5p in CSF exosomes (Gui et al. 2015), whereas another study showed a downregulation of miR-132-5p in *post mortem* CSF (Burgos et al. 2014).

More multicentric studies with larger cohorts, comparable specimens and techniques are needed to further evaluate miRNAs as putative biomarkers in PD.

miRNAs are also investigated as putative therapeutic targets. In a model of Huntington's disease (HD) both miR-132 strands were found to be decreased. Subsequently, after transduction of miR-132 with an adeno-associated virus (AAV), motor function improved, and lifespan expanded. Interestingly, the disease-causing *Huntingtin* (*HTT*) gene products were not changed. The authors discussed interactions of MECP2 and its binding to BDNF as a possible mechanistic background (Fukuoka et al. 2018; McFarland et al. 2014). In the R6/2 mouse model of HD miR-132-3p, miR-212-5p and miR-212-3p were found decreased and transduction with miR-132-3p overexpressing virus could even improve survival and motor symptoms (Fukuoka et al. 2018). Since the influence of miR-132/212 on neuroplasticity and learning was frequently described, they were also investigated in the context of AD. The knockdown of the miR-132/212 locus was found to impair learning, memory and tau metabolism – the pathological hallmark of AD (Smith et al. 2015; Leggio et al. 2017). In AD patients miR-132-3p was found downregulated and high miR-132/212 levels correlated with better cognitive scores which was associated with miR-132/212 induced downregulation of Sirtuin 1 (SIRT1) (Hadar et al. 2018). Another study observed an upregulation of miR-132/212 after acute and chronic stress in hippocampus or amygdala. Both, genetic overexpression and knockout of miR-132 increased anxiety-like behaviors (Aten et al. 2018).

In the context of PD, miR-132-3p directly targets the nuclear receptor related protein 1 (NURR1) and thereby inhibits the differentiation into mature dopaminergic neurons. As NURR1 regulates BDNF which in turn regulates miR-132, they jointly ensure their homeostasis (Yang et al. 2012; Lau et al. 2013; Heman-Ackah et al. 2013; Leggio et al. 2017). Mutations in NURR1 are also associated with familial Parkinsonism. It was reported to be downregulated in α-synuclein rich dopaminergic midbrain neurons of PD patients and deletion of NURR1 led to a progressive PD-like pathology. It is thus discussed as a putative target in PD treatment (Grimes et al. 2006; Lou and Liao 2012; Decressac et al. 2012; Decressac et al. 2013). In this specific context, PD patients would rather benefit from low levels of miR-132 to ensure stable levels of NURR1 whereas patients with other ND profit from increased miR-132 levels.

Several patents were already issued regarding therapeutic miRNAs (Chakraborty et al. 2017; Hesse and Arenz 2014). However, miRNAs are not yet approved as a therapeutic agent or medical target. Clinical trials are running for inhibitors and mimics of miRNAs in the treatment of scleroderma and different neoplasia. Two inhibitors of miR-122 against Hepatitis C even completed phase II trials (Rupaimoole and Slack 2017). Moreover, the discovery of non-coding RNAs led to the approval of the siRNA Patisiran for a rare type of hereditary polyneuropathy and various antisense oligonucleotides targeting diseases specific targets. Nusinersen (Spinraza) for patients with spinal muscle atrophy, eteplirsen (Exondys 51) in Duchenne muscle dystrophy and mipomersen (Kynamro) in homozygous familial hypocholesterolemia are the pioneers in this new field of therapeutic agents. More clinical trials are running for ALS targeting SOD1 and HD targeting HTT but not yet for PD – the second most common ND after AD (Khorkova and Wahlestedt 2017; Scoto et al. 2018; Hanna et al. 2019).

1.5 Aim of this study

Neuroscientific reports repeatedly reported beneficial effects of miR-132/212 expression for cognition and learning. Moreover, the miRNA cluster was investigated in various models of neurodegenerative diseases like HD, AD and also PD. In cell culture models of cortical, hippocampal, neuroblastoma and cell line neurons or embryonic stem cells molecular mechanisms were investigated and several targets of the miRNA cluster were identified (Hansen et al. 2016; Sun et al. 2018; Yang et al. 2012; Wanet et al. 2012). Single miRNA from the cluster were already explored in PD models (Fukuoka et al. 2018). However, their targets and mechanisms in dopaminergic midbrain neurons have not yet been investigated even though the degeneration of these neurons is an important part of PD pathophysiology. Most studies exclusively investigated effects of miR-132-3p but did not analyze other miRNA from the cluster nor combinations of them although they are transcribed together from a common gene locus. An upregulation of miR-132-3p and miR-212-3p was reported upon maturation in PMN. As mechanisms of neuronal maturation and growth are probably also relevant for neuronal regeneration, it is interesting to further investigate the effects of these miRNAs in these processes (Roser et al. 2018b).

This study aims to investigate the effects of increased levels of the mature strands miR-132-3p and miR-212-3p in PMN and *in vitro* models of PD. To increase miRNA levels, PMN are transfected with synthetic miRNA mimics. In a second step, the underlying mechanisms of miR-132-3p- or miR-212-3p-mediated effects are investigated. In contrast to most other studies, experiments are performed for both mature miRNAs to compare their effects. Moreover, a combined condition with increased levels of both miRNAs is included. Based on the observed effects and identified mechanisms the therapeutic potential of the two miRNAs is evaluated.

First, an optimal concentration for the transfection with synthetic miRNA mimics had to be found. Subsequently, the influence of increased miR-132-3p or miR-212-3p levels on neurite outgrowth in dopaminergic PMN was analyzed. To investigate possible effects on neuroregeneration and neuroprotection a mechanical and a toxic degeneration model were used. For an unbiased investigation of protein alterations induced by increased levels of the miRNA, the PMN's proteome was assessed by liquid chromatography with tandem mass spectrometry (LC/MS/MS) for an identification and quantification of its proteins (proteomics). Analysis of the proteome can both help to identify new targets but also to reveal indirect or downstream effects of the transfected miRNA. Selected proteins from literature and proteomics analysis were also investigated by immunoblotting.

2 Material

2.1 Reagents

Table 2 Table of reagents used for experiments

Reagent	Producer	Purpose
1-bromo-3-chloropropane	Sigma Aldrich (Germany)	RNA isolation from PMN
1-methyl-4-phenylpyridinium (MPP^+)	Sigma Aldrich (Germany)	PD in vitro model in PMN
2-propanol	AppliChem (Germany)	RNA isolation, SDS gel protection
4',6-diamidino-2-phenylindole (DAPI)	Sigma Aldrich (Germany)	Nuclear co-staining for ICC
Acrylamide	AppliChem (Germany)	Gel preparation for SDS-PAGE
Ammonium chloride (NH_4Cl)	Merck (Germany)	Fixation for staining
Ammonium persulfate (APS)	Sigma Aldrich (Germany)	Gel polymerization for SDS-PAGE
B-27 Supplement	Gibco (Germany)	Supplement for cell culture medium
Bovine serum albumin (BSA, 2mg/ml)	AppliChem (Germany)	BCA measurement of protein concentration
Bromophenol blue	Sigma Aldrich (Germany)	Stacking gel
cOmplete Protease Inhibitor	Sigma Aldrich (Germany)	Laemmli buffer supplement
DAKO antibody diluent	DAKO (Germany)	Staining solutions for ICC
DNAse	Sigma Aldrich (Germany)	Cell culture processing
Fetal calf serum (FCS)	Biochrom (Germany)	Cell culture processing
Glycoblue Coprecipitant	Thermo Fisher Scientific (USA)	RNA isolation
Hank's Balanced Salt Solution (HBSS)	Gibco (Germany)	CMF for cell culture
Laminin	Sigma Aldrich (Germany)	Well/ coverslip coating
L-Ascrobic acid (L-AA)	Sigma Aldrich (Germany)	Cell culture medium
L-Glutamine 200mM (100x)	Gibco (Germany)	Cell culture medium
Methanol	AppliChem (Germany)	Transfer buffer for Western blot
Mowiol	Sigma Aldrich (Germany)	Mounting of coverslips
Neurobasal A medium	Gibco (Germany)	Cell culture medium
Non-fat dried milk	AppliChem (Germany)	Blocking and antibody dilution for Western blot
Paraformaldehyde (PFA)	AppliChem (Germany)	Fixation for staining
Phosphate buffered saline (PBS)	AppliChem (Germany)	Washing of samples
PhosStop	Roche (Germany)	Laemmli buffer supplement
Pierce BCA Assay Reagent A + B	Thermo Fisher Scientific (USA)	Measurement of protein concentration

Reagent	Producer	Purpose
Poly-L-ornithine (PLO)	Sigma Aldrich (Germany)	Coating of cell culture wells or coverslips
Precision Plus Protein Dual Color	Bio-Rad (Germany)	Protein size reference in during Western blot
Radioimmunoprecipitation (RIPA) buffer	Thermo Fisher Scientific (USA)	Cell lysis
RNAse free (DEPC treated) water	Sigma Aldrich (Germany)	Dilution of RNA or DNA
Sodium dodecyl sulfate (SDS)	AppliChem (Germany	Laemmli Buffer, SDS-PAGE
Tetramethyl-ethylenediamine (TEMED)	Roth (Germany)	Gel Polymerization for SDS-PAGE
Tris HCl	AppliChem (Germany)	Preparing TBS for Western blot
TritonX 100	AppliChem (Germany)	Permeabilization for ICC staining
Trizol (TRI Reagent)	Sigma Aldrich (Germany)	Cell lysis for RNA isolation
Trypsin	Biochrom (Germany)	Processing tissue for PMN
Tween 20	AppliChem (Germany)	Washing detergent for Western blot

2.2 Primers, miRNA mimics and kits

Table 3 Table of primers, miRNA mimics, their sequences and kits used for experiments

Kit / Sequence	Producer	Purpose
AllStars Negative Control siRNA (20nM)	Qiagen (Germany)	Transfection of PMN
ECL Prime Western blotting Detection Reagent	GE Healthcare (UK)	Western blot
HiPerfect transfection reagent	Qiagen (Germany)	Transfection of PMN
Hs_RNU6-2_11 miScript Primer Assay	Qiagen (Germany)	qPCR
miScript II RT Kit Qiagen	Qiagen (Germany)	Reverse Transcription
miScript SYBR Green PCR Kit	Qiagen (Germany)	qPCR
Mm_miR-212 miScript Primer Assay	Qiagen (Germany)	qPCR
Syn-mmu-miR-129-2-3p (AAGCCCUUACCCCAAAAAGCAU-3p)	Qiagen (Germany)	Transfection of PMN
Syn-mmu-miR-132-3p (UAACAGUCUACAGCCAUGGUCG-3p)	Qiagen (Germany)	Transfection of PMN
Syn-mmu-miR-212-3p (UAACAGUCUCCAGUCACGGCCA-3p)	Qiagen (Germany)	Transfection of PMN
Syn-mmu-miR-7b-5p (UGGAAGACUUGUGAUUUUGUUGUU-5p)	Qiagen (Germany)	Transfection of PMN

2.3 Antibodies

Table 4 Table of antibodies and their dilution used for immunocytochemistry

Primary Antibodies	Producer	Dilution
Anti-tyrosine hydroxylase (anti-TH) – polyclonal, anti-rabbit	Zytomed (Germany)	1:1000 in DAKO antibody diluent
Secondary Antibodies	**Producer**	**Dilution**
Goat IgG anti-rabbit IgG, Cy3 conjugated	Cell Signaling (United Kingdom)	1:250 in DAKO antibody diluent

Table 5 Table of antibodies and their dilutions used for immunoblotting

Primary Antibodies	Producer	Dilution
Anti-EPHA5 – polyclonal, rabbit	LSBio (USA)	1:1000 in 5 % milk TBS-T
Anti-GAPDH – monoclonal, mouse	HyTest Ltd (Finland)	1:5000 in 2.5 % milk TBS-T
Anti-MECP2 – monoclonal, rabbit	Cell Signaling Technology (USA)	1:1000 in 5 % BSA TBS-T
Anti-ROCK2 – monoclonal, rabbit	Cell Signaling Technology (USA)	1:1000 in 5 % BSA-TBS-T
Anti-TAX1BP3 – monoclonal, rabbit	Abcam (UK)	1:1500 in 5 % BSA-TBS-T
ARHGAP32 (p250GAP) antiserum, rabbit	Dr. Takanobu Nakazawa, Institute of Medical Science, University of Tokyo, Tokyo, Japan (Nakazawa et al. 2003)	1:800 in 2.5 % milk-TBS-T
Secondary Antibodies	**Producer**	**Dilution**
Anti-mouse IgG, HRP linked Antibody	Cell Signaling Technology (USA)	1:2000 in 2.5 % milk TBS-T
Anti-rabbit IgG, HRP-linked Antibody	Cell Signaling Technology (USA)	1:1000 in 5 % milk TBS-T

2.4 Solutions and buffers

Table 6 Table of solutions and buffers used for experiments

Solution	Composition	Purpose
Blocking solution for Western blot	5 % non-fat dried milk in TBS-T	Prevents unspecific binding in Western blot experiments
Borate buffer	boric acid buffered with NaOH to pH 8.4	Dilution of PLO
Calcium-magnesium-free medium (CMF)	10 % HBSS diluted in distilled water, pH adjusted with ~ sodium bicarbonate	PMN preparation and cell processing
Cell culture medium	2 % B27-supplement, 1 % glutamine, 0.1 % 200mM L-AA in Neurobasal	PMN cell culture
DAPI solution	1 µg/ ml DAPI in PBS	Nuclear staining for ICC
Laemmli buffer	312.5 mM Tris pH 6.8, 10 % SDS, 50 % Glycerin, 0.005 % Bromophenol blue, 100 mM DTT	Protein solution for SDS-PAGE
Phosphate buffered saline	0.1 % TritonX 100 in PBS	Permeabilization of cells for ICC
Tris	10 mM Tris-buffered saline pH 8.0	Dilution of reagents for Western blot
Tris buffered saline (TBS)	10 mM Tris HCl, 150 mM NaCl in distilled water	Dilution of reagents for Western blot
Tris buffered saline with Tween20 (TBS-T)	0.1 % Tween20 in TBS, pH 7.6	Dilution of reagents for Western blot

2.5 Composition of gels for SDS-PAGE

Table 7 Composition of gels for SDS-PAGE

Compounds	8 % gel	14 % gel	Stacking gel
30% acrylamide	2.27 ml	3.97 ml	0.325 ml
4x Tris Cl/SDS pH 8.8	2.13 ml	2.13 ml	----
4x Tris Cl/SDS pH 6.8	---	---	0.625 ml
water (distilled)	4.11 ml	2.41 ml	1.515 ml
10% APS	42.5 µl	42.5 µl	12.5 µl
TEMED	4.25 µl	4.25 µl	2.5 µl
0.5% Bromophenol blue	---	---	10 µl

(Composition for two gels)

2.6 Equipment

Table 8 Table of equipment used for experiments

Equipment	Producer	Purpose
12 well cell culture plates	Sarstedt (Germany)	PMN culture for RNA isolation
24 well cell culture plates CytoOne	USA Scientific (USA)	PMN culture for ICC
6 well cell culture plates Cellstar	Greiner bio-one (Austria)	PMN culture for protein isolation
96 well micro test plates	Sarstedt (Germany)	BCA measurement of protein concentration
96 well microamp Endura Plate	Thermo Fisher Scientific (USA)	qPCR
Cover slides 76 x 26 mm	Menzel (Germany)	PMN culture for ICC
EV 2310 power supply	Consort (Belgium)	Power supply for Western blot and SDS PAGE
Fusion Pulse Chemiluminescence Imager	Vilber Lourmat (Germany)	Western blot Imaging
Mastercylcer nexus X2	Eppendorf (Germany	Reverse Transcription
Micro-centrifuge 5415R	Eppendorf (Germany)	Cell culture Processing
Mini-Protean Tetra-Cell system	Bio-Rad (Germany)	Western blot and SDS PAGE
NanoDrop One	Thermo Fisher Scientific (USA)	Measuring RNA concentration and purity
Polyvinylidene fluoride (PVDF) immunoblotting membrane	GE Healthcare (United Kingdom)	Western blot
Quant Studio 3	Thermo Fisher Scientific (USA)	q-RT-PCR machine control
RNAse -Exitus Plus	AppliChem (Germany)	Cleaning before RNA work
Spacer plates / short plates	Bio-Rad (Germany)	Preparing gels for SDS-Page
Tecan Spark 10M plate reader	Tecan (Switzerland)	BCA measurement of protein concentration
Thermomixer Comfort	Eppendorf (Germany)	Sample boiling and incubation

2.7 Software

Table 9 Table of software used for experiments, data analysis and figure design

Equipment	Producer	Purpose
AxioVision 4.6 Software	Carl Zeiss (Germany)	Microscope control
CorelDraw X6 16.1.0.843 Graphics Suite	Corel Corporation (Canada)	Figure design
Evolution Capt 17.03	Vilber Lourmat, (Germany)	Imaging of immunoblots and image analysis
GraphPad Prism 5.04	GraphPad software (USA)	Graph design and statistical analysis
ImageJ 1.51	National Institute of Health (USA)	Neurite tracing and somata counting
KyPlot 5.0	KyensLab (Japan)	Statistical analysis
Neuron J Plugin 1.4.3	Erik Meijering (Netherlands)	Neurite tracing
Perseus 1.5.6.0	Computational Systems Biochemistry, Max Planck Institute, Martinsried Germany (Tyanova et al. 2016)	LC/MS/MS SWATH data evaluation
Venny 2.1 (Web tool)	Juan Carlos Oliveros, Centro Nacional de Biotechnologia (Spain)	Overlap analysis for proteomics data

3 Methods

3.1 Primary midbrain neuronal cultures

3.1.1 Experimental animals

Pregnant C57Bl6/J mice were used as donor animals for primary cell culture preparation. They were provided by the central animal facility of the University Medical Center of Göttingen. The mice were kept in standard multiple housing in 12 hours dark/light cycle and were fed *ad libitum*. At the embryonic day 12.5 shortly before preparation, they were euthanized using carbon dioxide (CO_2) and death was confirmed by testing the mice's toe pain reflexes. All experiments are in line with the national German animal protection law and were approved by the local authorities (project name: T10/28 Embryonenentnahme).

3.1.2 Coating the coverslips and culture plates

To provide suitable growing conditions for the PMN cultures, wells were coated with poly-L-ornithine (PLO) dissolved in borate buffer and diluted with sterile water to a final concentration of 0.1 mg/ml incubating overnight at room temperature (RT). Subsequently, wells were coated with laminin (0.1 μg/ml) diluted in neurobasal medium (Gibco, Germany) without supplements, incubated for one hour at 37°C / 5 % CO_2 and stored at 4°C. For immunocytochemistry (ICC) cleaned and sterilized glass coverslips (Ø 12 mm) were placed into wells of a 24 well-plate and coated as described above. Shortly before preparation, the laminin solution was removed, wells were washed three times with neurobasal medium (free of supplements) and the required amount of supplemented neurobasal medium (2 % B27, 1 % glutamine, 0.1 % 200 mM L-ascorbic acid (L-AA)) was filled in every well (Table 10).

3.1.3 Preparation of primary midbrain neurons

The euthanized, pregnant mice were disinfected with 70 % ethanol and skinned using two small Overholt forceps. Afterwards the peritoneum was opened, and the uterus was worked free from ligaments, vessels and the vagina. Embryos were then removed from their amniotic sacs and kept in ice-cold calcium-magnesium-free medium (CMF). Subsequently, the midbrain vesicle was dissected and opened longitudinally on its dorsal part. Meninges were removed and the ventral part of the midbrain vesicle containing the dopaminergic neurons was dissected and kept in ice-cold CMF. Cells were centrifuged at 1000 rounds per minute (equal to 86 x g relative centrifugal force (rcf)) for 1 min, CMF was removed, and the tissue was kept for 12 minutes in a 37°C water bath with 0.25 % trypsin for tissue digestion. Afterwards, 50 µl DNAse (5 mg/ml) was added and the cell suspension was again centrifuged at 1000 rounds per minute (rpm) / 86 x g rcf for 1 min. Trypsin was removed, and fetal calf serum (FCS) was added to inactivate trypsin. To achieve a single cell suspension, the solution was triturated with a very narrow, fire polished Pasteur pipette. After a final centrifugation at 1000 rpm / 86 x g rcf for 4 min, CMF was removed, and the cells were resuspended in supplemented pre-warmed neurobasal medium. Concentration of healthy cells was quantified using a Neubauer chamber and plated accordingly as displayed in Table 10. The cell cultures were then kept in a humidified incubator at 37°C and 5 % CO_2. If the cells were kept until DIV 4, half of the wells total medium was changed at DIV 3. This protocol for PMN cell culture was established earlier in the same lab and was shown to contain on average ~ 6 % dopaminergic neurons, 94 % gamma-aminobutyric acid (GABA) transmitting neurons and only single cells positive for glial fibrillary acid protein (GFAP) (Lingor et al. 1999).

Table 10 Number of cells and amount of medium for different cell culture plates and experiments

Wells per plate	Number of cells	Final amount of medium	Purpose
6 wells	3 x 10^6	2400 µl	Preparation for protein isolation
12 wells	1.5 x 10^6	1200 µl	Preparation for RNA isolation
24 wells	650.000	600 µl	Preparation for ICC experiments

3.2 Transfection of PMN cultures with miRNA mimics

Cell cultures were always transfected at DIV 1, 24 hours after plating the cells. The transfection solution was based on supplemented cell culture medium, complemented with 2 µl HiPerfect transfection reagent (Qiagen, Germany) per 100 µl transfection solution and the respective miRNA mimics (Qiagen, Germany). The miRNA mimics are transfected as double stranded synthetic RNA, being only one strand biologically active according to the manufacturer. AllStars Negative Control siRNA (Qiagen, Germany) – a validated negative control which has no homology to any mammalian gene known – was used as negative control (NC). The amount of miRNA mimics respectively NC siRNA was calculated for concentrations of 0.5 nM, 5 nM or 50 nM for the corresponding final volume of the well depending on the plate format (Table 10). Before adding to the plates, the transfection solution was vortexed for 1 min and left undisturbed for 10 min at RT to allow formation of transfection complexes. Three hours after transfection, half of the culture media was removed from the wells and replaced with prewarmed supplemented cell culture medium.

3.3 Measuring miRNA levels for transfection amount study

To find a suitable amount for the transfection of PMN with miRNA mimics three different concentrations of 0.5 nM, 5 nM and 50 nM were tested. All RNA work was performed under laminar air flow after cleaning thoroughly with RNAseZAP. Earlier studies from the lab demonstrated that the transfection protocol successfully transfects 84 ± 1.0 % of all PMN cells (Roser et al. 2018b). For the miR-132-3p the transfection efficacy and dose findings experiments were performed by L. Caldi Gomes in a previous project using the same protocol (Caldi Gomes 2016).

3.3.1 RNA Isolation from PMN cultures

Total RNA was isolated from PMN at DIV 3. At first, all the media was removed, and cells were washed once with cold *phosphate buffered saline* (PBS). Afterwards, cells were lysed with 1 ml Trizol reagent (Sigma Aldrich, Germany) per well incubating for 5 min at RT. The lysate was pipetted up and down several times and transferred to an Eppendorf tube. For phase separation, 100 µl of 1-bromo-3-chlor-propane were added to each tube, mixed thoroughly and kept undisturbed for 5 min at RT. After 15 min centrifugation with 12.000 x g rcf at 4°C, the upper – RNA containing – layer was carefully transferred to another Eppendorf tube, without entering or disturbing the other layers. For RNA precipitation, 500 µl isopropanol were added together with 1.5 µl Glycoblue (Thermo Fisher Scientific, USA) to stain the RNA pellet and cells were kept overnight at -20°C. The next day, samples were centrifuged for 30 min at 12.000 x g rcf at 4°C. Isopropanol was removed and the blue colored RNA pellet was washed two times with cold 75 % ethanol – carefully watching not to break the pellet. In between two washing steps, samples were centrifuged 5 min at 12.000 x g rcf at 4°C, before the ethanol was removed again. After removing the ethanol, the second time, pellets were air dried for 12 min and then diluted in 10 to 15 µl RNAse free water. Finally, samples were incubated 5 min at 55°C (Thermomix comfort, Eppendorf, Germany), to completely dissolve all RNA. Afterwards, samples were stored at -20°C.

3.3.2 RNA and DNA quantification

To measure the total concentration of the isolated RNA and to exclude possible contaminations with extraction liquids or proteins, 1 µl of the RNA sample was pipetted into the measuring unit of the Nano Drop One device (Thermo Fisher Scientific). After the reverse transcription the concentration of the complementary DNA (cDNA) was also measured with the Nano Drop One device.

3.3.3 Reverse transcription

In a first step, RNA had to be converted into cDNA. The concentration measured in the NanoDrop One was used to dilute 500 ng RNA in 6 µl RNAse free water. A Master Mix was prepared as shown in Table 11 containing miScript HiSpec Buffer, Nucleics Mix and Reverse Transcriptase (all Qiagen, Germany). All pipetting was done under RNAse free conditions. Afterwards, everything incubated in the Mastercylcer nexus X2 (Eppendorf, Germany) at 37°C for 60 minutes, followed by 5 minutes at 95°C to inactivate the enzyme. The concentration of the produced cDNA was also measured using the NanoDrop One device. Subsequently, samples were stored at -20°C.

Table 11 Master Mix contaminants for reverse transcription

Component	Volume per reaction
500 ng Sample RNA diluted in 6 µl RNase-free water	6 µl
5x miScript HiSpec Buffer	2 µl
10x miScript Nucleics Mix	1 µl
miScript Reverse Transcriptase	1 µl
Total	10 µl per reaction

3.3.4 Quantitative real time polymerase chain reaction

The amount of cDNA gained from the isolated RNA after reverse transcription was assessed by quantitative real-time polymerase chain reaction (q-RT-PCR) using the QuantStudio 3 q-RT-PCR machine (Thermo Fisher Scientific, USA). The small nuclear RNA U6-2 gene (RNU6-2) was selected as housekeeping control gene. First, a Master Mix was prepared for every target gene as displayed in Table 12.

Table 12 Master Mix contaminants for qPCR

Components	Volume per reaction
2x QuantiTect SYBR Green PCR Master Mix	7.5 µl
10x miScript Universal Primer	1.5 µl
10x miScript Specific Primer (RNU6-2 or miR-212)	1.5 µl
RNAse-free water	3.0 µl
Total Volume Master Mix per reaction	13.5 µl

Afterwards, 1.5 µl of the sample cDNA was pipetted to the wells on a 96-well-plate, followed by 13.5 µl Master Mix. All experimental conditions (three different concentrations of miRNA mimics, NC siRNA and the respective corresponding RNU-6 control) were measured in duplicates on the same plate. The plate was sealed and centrifuged 2 min at 1000 rpm / 86 x g rcf and loaded into the RT-PCR machine. The qPCR settings are displayed in Table 13.

Table 13 Cycle length and temperature for qPCR

Step	Time	Temperature
PCR initial activation step	15 min	95°C
3-step cycling		
Denaturation	15 s	94°C
Annealing	30 s	55°C
Extension	30 s	70°C
Number of cycles	40 cycles	

The q-RT-PCR measurements were only taken into consideration as long as two blank samples of each Master Mix with 1.5 µl of the used water did not show any contamination. The delta-delta cycle threshold method (ΔΔCt method) was used to quantify the expression data of the mRNA. The Ct values of miRNA were first normalized to the RNU6-2 Ct values from the same sample and subsequently to the experimental NC siRNA transfected cells.

3.4 Neurodegeneration models *in vitro*

In order to investigate the influence of the experimental conditions on neuroprotection, neurodegeneration and regeneration of dopaminergic PMN, two cell stress models were used.

3.4.1 Scratch lesion model

To simulate a mechanical damage model, cultures were scratched twice in an X-shape with a sterile 200 µl pipette at DIV 2. As in all experiments for ICC, the cultures were fixated at DIV 4, followed by ICC staining and imaging. For this experiment, two cultures treated with 5 nM miR-132-3p were prepared, stained and imaged by L. Caldi Gomes following the same protocol as described here. The subsequent evaluation was performed together with all other conditions.

3.4.2 1-Methyl-4-phenylpyridinium (MPP^+) treatment

Stress resistance and neuroprotective abilities were investigated using MPP^+ which specifically targets dopaminergic neurons through catecholaminergic transporters. Within the cell, MPP^+ can generate free radicals, disturb calcium homeostasis, axonal transport and inhibit mitochondrial complex I. This can lead to insufficient energy supply and induction of apoptosis (Kopin 1992).

Cell survival was investigated in PMN on 24 well-plates with coverslips. The MPP^+ treatment was applied at DIV 2 at a final concentration of 2 µM per well, diluted in prewarmed supplemented cell culture medium. As vehicle control, duplicates of every experimental condition were treated with prewarmed, supplemented cell culture media instead of MPP^+. The whole medium of all wells was removed and replaced with prewarmed supplemented neurobasal medium to avoid augmented toxicity 24 hours later. Cells were fixated at DIV 4 and prepared for immunocytochemistry. For this experiment, three 5 nM miR-132-3p treated PMN cultures, were prepared, MPP^+ treated, stained and imaged by L. Caldi Gomes following the same protocol. The subsequent evaluation was performed together with all other conditions.

3.5 Immunocytochemistry

The influence of the transfected miRNA mimics on neurite growth or regeneration of dopaminergic PMN was evaluated using immunocytochemistry.

3.5.1 Fixation, staining and preparation for immunocytochemistry of PMN

Cells for ICC were always fixated at DIV 4 using 350 µl of 4 % paraformaldehyde (PFA) per well incubating for 20 min at RT. Afterwards, PFA was removed and 350 µl of 200 mM ammonium chloride (NH_4Cl) were added incubating 10 min followed by three times washing for 5 min with PBS. If staining was not performed the same day, cells were stored sufficiently covered with PBS at 4°C. For permeabilization, cells were incubated 10 min with PBS-T (PBS with 0.1 % Triton) and blocked with DAKO antibody diluent for 20 minutes. A primary rabbit antibody against tyrosine hydroxylase (TH, Zytomed) was used to selectively stain dopaminergic neurons. For this purpose, the primary antibody was diluted 1:1000 in DAKO antibody diluent and incubated for 1 h at 37°C with 180 µl per well. After three more times washing with PBS for 5 min, a secondary Cy3 conjugated goat anti-rabbit antibody, diluted 1:250 was applied incubating 30 min at 37°C. Once more, cells were washed three times for 5 min with PBS and 200 µl of 4',6-diamidino-2-phenylindole (DAPI) (1 µg/ml in PBS) was applied for 5 min for a nuclear co-staining. After washing the cells three more times for 5 min with PBS, coverslips were mounted on glass slides using prewarmed Mowiol. If not described differently all incubation and washing steps were performed on a shaker at RT, protected from light.

3.5.2 Immunocytochemistry imaging

The coverslips were imaged at 20x magnification using the Axioplan 2 imaging microscope (Zeiss, Germany) together with the corresponding AxioVision 40 software (Version 4.8.2.0). For evaluation of neurite growth and MPP^+ survival, four by four mosaic images were taken at prior defined spots 2500 µm towards the center from three, six, nine and twelve o'clock sides of the coverslips. For the scratch lesion experiment, four by six mosaic images were taken along the scratch border. During one experiment all microscope and software settings were always kept unchanged.

3.5.3 Evaluation of immunocytochemistry photomicrographs

To evaluate the neurite growth of dopaminergic PMN, all TH positive neurites detectable in the Cy3 channel were quantified using the Neuron J Plugin of the Image J software (version 1.4.3). Subsequently, the total number of TH positive somata was counted with Image J (version 1.51) and an average neurite length per soma was calculated. In the scratch lesion experiment, only the length of regenerating TH positive neurites from the scratch border to the neurite tip was measured. Afterwards, the sum of the length of the seven longest neurites in each picture was calculated for normalization. For the evaluation of neuroprotective effects of the miRNA mimics in the MPP^+ model, TH positive cell somata were counted and divided by the numbers in the medium treated vehicle control of the same condition. During one experiment, the defined scale and magnification were always kept the same. All images were analyzed at the same monitor in a darkened room.

3.6 Proteome analysis of miRNA transfected PMN

To identify proteins regulated by the transfected miRNA mimics, proteins were isolated from PMN and subjected to mass spectrometry for a first and unbiased screening. Selected proteins were then further evaluated using Western blot.

3.6.1 Preparation of cell lysates from PMN

Cell lysates were always prepared at DIV 3. To reduce cell metabolism, all steps were performed on ice and with cold reagents. First, media was removed, and dead cells were washed out with PBS. Subsequently, 100 µl radioimmunoprecipitation assay (RIPA) buffer (Thermo Fisher Scientific, USA) supplemented with phosphatase inhibitor 1:20 and complete proteasome inhibitor 1:20 were given to every well and incubated 10 min on ice. Subsequently, cells were scraped off using a cell scraper and transferred to Eppendorf tubes.

Afterwards, all samples were sonicated two times for 15 s at an amplitude of 40 % resulting in an additional mechanical cell lysis. Samples were kept on ice between sonication cycles to avoid protein denaturation.

3.6.2 Protein quantification and processing of cell lysates

To prepare samples with equal protein concentrations for further experiments, the protein concentration was measured with the Pierce bicinchoninic acid Assay (Pierce BCA Assay, Thermo Fisher Scientific, USA). Triplicates of 1 µl per sample diluted in 199 µl BCA reagent (Reagent B: Reagent A, 1:50) were compared to an eight well standard curve. The standard curve had 20 µg of bovine serum albumin (BSA 2 mg/ml, AppliChem, Germany) in its first well, subsequently diluted 1:2 to the next wells (BSA per well: 20 µg, 10 µg, 5 µg, 2.5 µg, 1.25 µg, 0.625 µg, 0.313 µg, 0.156 µg) and filled up to 200 µl BCA solution per well. All samples and standard curve wells were run in triplicates and incubated for 30 min at 37°C. Finally, absorbance was measured at 562 nm using the Tecan Spark 10M plate reader (Tecan, Switzerland) and concentration was calculated relatively to the standard curve. Subsequently, a solution of the required protein concentration diluted in Laemmli buffer with 10 % dithiothreitol (DTT) was prepared and incubated 5 min at 95°C before storing at -80°C.

3.6.3 LC/MS/MS on PMN protein lysates

For every experimental condition three replicates per condition á 50 µg in 30 µl Laemmli buffer with 10 % DTT were prepared as described above. The following protein analysis by LC/MS/MS was performed by the proteomics facility led by Dr. Christof Lenz and Prof. Dr. Henning Urlaub, Institute of Clinical Chemistry, University Medical Center Göttingen who kindly provided the following protocol. The material used for the LC/MS/MS is not listed in the material chapter of this book.

In a first step, sodium dodecyl sulfate (SDS) was removed by running 50 µg of each sample on 4-12 % NuPAGE Novex Bis-Tris Minigels (Invitrogen, USA) for 1.5 cm. The protein bands were stained using Coomassie, cut out, treated with DTT for reduction, iodacetamide for alkylation and finally with trypsin overnight for in-gel digestion. After the solution had dried in a Speedvac, samples were stored at -20°C (Atanassov and Urlaub 2013).

Library preparation was performed from a pool of all samples (total amount: 80 µg) after separation into eight fractions using a reversed phase spin column (Pierce High pH Reversed-Phase Peptide Fractionation Kit, Thermo Fisher Scientific, USA). A synthetic peptide standard was used for retention time alignment (iRT standard, Biognosys, Switzerland).

Prior to the mass spectrometry run, peptides were dissolved to a concentration of 0.3 µg/µl in loading buffer (2 % acetonitrile, 0.1 % formic acid in water). On a precolumn (0.18 mm ID x 20 mm, Symmetry C18, 5 µm, Waters, USA) 1.5 µg digested protein were enriched for each analysis and separated on an analytical RP-C18 column (0.075 mm ID x 250 mm, HSS T3, 1.8 µm, Waters, USA) using a 90 min linear gradient of 5-35 % acetonitrile/0.1 % formic acid at 300 nl min^{-1}. Finally, protein digests were than conducted to a nanoflow chromatography system (Eksigent nanoLC425) hyphenated to a hybrid triple quadrupole-TOF mass spectrometer (TripleTOF 5600+) equipped with a Nanospray III ion source (Ionspray Voltage 2400 V, Interface Heater Temperature 150°C, Sheath Gas Setting 12) under control of Analyst TF 1.7.1 (all AB Sciex, USA).

A Top25 data-dependent acquisition method was used for qualitative LC/MS/MS analysis. The total cycle time was 2.9 s with an MS survey scan of *m/z* 350 - 1250 for 350 ms at a resolution of 30,000 full width at half maximum (FWHM) and following MS/MS scans of *m/z* 180 - 1600 for 100 ms at 17,500 FWHM. The precursor isolation width was 0.7 FWHM. Only precursors with charge states of 2+, 3+, and 4+ with an MS intensity of at least 125 counts per second were selected for MS/MS. The MS/MS run was started by collision induced dissociation with nitrogen as a collision gas at the manufacturer's default rolling collision energy settings with a dynamic exclusion time of 30 s. For one reversed phase fraction four technical replicates were analyzed to construct a spectral library.

In 65 variable size windows between 400 - 1,050 *m/z* range MS/MS data were acquired for data independent quantitative sequential windowed acquisition of all theoretical fragment ion mass spectra (SWATH-MS) analysis (Zhang et al. 2015). Rolling collision energy settings for charge state 2+ were used for fragmentation. A 100 ms survey scan and fragment acquisition for 40 ms per segment at an *m/z* range of 350 - 1400 led to an overall cycle time of 2.75 s.

For protein identification, the total MS/MS spectra from the combined qualitative analysis was compared against 52 laboratory contaminants and the UniProtKB *Mus musculus* reference proteome (revision 12-2017, 60,769 entries) using the ProteinPilot software version 5.0 (AB Sciex, USA) at "thorough" settings. Retention time was corrected by the iRT standard and linked to the MS/MS library at F (FDR) of 1%.

Subsequently, the spectral library was generated, and SWATH-peaks extracted using the SWATH quantitation microAPP (version 2.0) of the PeakView software (version 2.1, AB Sciex, USA). Only proteins detected in every run and sample were taken into consideration for quantification (Lambert et al. 2013; Losensky et al. 2017). Peak areas were summed to peptide, and finally protein area values.

3.6.4 Interpretation of SWATH-MS data and miRNA target prediction

For statistical analysis data were imported to Perseus 1.5.6.0 software, quantitative values were log_2 transformed to achieve a normal data distribution and Perseus' Significance B analysis was performed (Cox and Mann 2008; Tyanova et al. 2016). Subsequently, the significantly regulated proteins were imported to the Database for Annotation Visualization, and Integrated Discovery (DAVID, version 6.8) for KEGG pathway and gene ontology (GO) analysis (Huang et al. 2007; Huang et al. 2009).

In order to identify predicted targets among the regulated proteins in SWATH-MS, target prediction was performed with three different target prediction algorithms – targetscan.org (Agarwal et al. 2015), microrna.org (Betel et al. 2010; Betel et al. 2008) and mirwalk.org (Dweep and Gretz 2015). Whereas microrna.org and mirwalk.org differentiate between miR-132-3p and miR-212-3p, tragetscan.org predicts targets only based on the seed sequence which is the same for miR-132-3p and miR-212-3p. Comparative analysis of predicted targets and proteins measured in SWATH MS was performed with Venny 2.1.0 (Oliveros 2007).

3.6.5 Western blot

In a first step of cell lysate analysis, proteins were separated by SDS-polyacrylamide gel electrophoresis (SDS-PAGE). The anionic SDS contained in the Laemmli buffer covers the amino acids of proteins so that all proteins become similarly negatively charged and are only separated according to their size and molecular weight. Furthermore, the gels basic pH of 8.8 reduces positive protein charges. According to the BCA measurements, stock solutions of 1.25 µg/µl in Laemmli Buffer with 10 % DTT were prepared for every sample. The electrophoresis was run with 25 µg per sample. For band identification 4 µl marker (Precision Plus Protein Dual Color, Bio-Rad, Germany) were used. Electrophoresis was run in a Mini-Protean Tetra-Cell system (Bio-Rad, Germany) until the running had reached the bottom of the gel.

Subsequently to the SDS-PAGE, the separated proteins were transferred to a polyvinylidene fluoride (PVDF) membrane (GE Healthcare, United Kingdome). First, the PVDF membrane was incubated in pure methanol for 30 s and then packed in the same system as used for electrophoresis. The proteins were transferred in transfer buffer containing 10 % methanol at constant voltage and 4°C. Afterwards, the membrane was incubated in 5 % non-fat dried milk (AppliChem, Germany) diluted in tris buffered saline with Tween20 (TBS-T) followed by the incubation with the required primary antibody overnight at 4°C.

Afterwards, the membrane was washed three times with TBS-T for 10 minutes and an appropriate secondary antibody incubated one hour at RT on the shaker followed by three more times washing with TBS-T for 10 minutes.

For three proteins the SDS-PAGE was run on 8 % gels at 40 V for 4.5 hours followed by 16 hours transfer at 30 V using the following antibodies: anti-ROCK2 (Rho associated coiled-coil containing protein kinase 2) rabbit antibody (1:1000 in 5 % BSA in TBS-T), anti-EPHA5 (EPH-Receptor A5) rabbit antibody (1:1000 in 5 % milk in TBS-T, LS Bio, USA), anti-ARHGAP32 (Rho GTPases activating protein 32) rabbit-antiserum (1:800 in 2.5 % milk in TBS-T by Takanobu Nakazawa, Tokyo, Japan (Nakazawa et al. 2003)). Two more proteins were investigated on 14 % gels with an electrophoresis at 80 V for 2.5 hours, followed by two hours transfer at 100 V with the following antibodies: anti-MECP2 monoclonal rabbit antibody (1:1000 in 5% BSA in TBS-T, Cell signaling technology, UK), anti-TAX1BP3 (Tax1 binding protein 3) monoclonal rabbit antibody (1:1500, in 5 % BSA in TBST-T, Abcam, UK). The gel composition can be found in the material chapter (Table 7). In all experiments, GAPDH was used as loading control (1:5000 in 2.5 % milk in TBS-T, HyTest Ltd, Finland). As secondary antibodies, horseradish-peroxidase (HRP)-linked anti-rabbit IgG (1:1000 in 5 % milk in TBS-T, Cell signaling, UK) and anti-mouse IgG (1:2000 in 2.5 % milk in TBS-T, Cell signaling, UK) were used.

Finally, the blot was imaged using the Fusion Pulse Chemiluminescence Imager (Vilber, Germany) with ECL Prime Western blotting Detection Reagent (GE Healthcare, United Kingdom) controlled by the EvolutionCapt 17.03 software. Also, the image analysis was performed with the named software.

3.7 Statistical analysis

KyPlot v2.0 (KyensLab) and Prism v5.04 (GraphPad software) were used for statistical analysis and graph design. Data were tested for normal distribution using the Shapiro-Wilk test and are given as mean or median ± standard error of the mean (SEM, always given with the figure description). A pair-wise comparison of normally distributed date was performed with a one-way analysis of variance (ANOVA) followed by Tukey's test for the interpretation of qPCR data. All other experiments compared more than one experimental condition to NC. Therefore, a one-way ANOVA followed by Dunnett's test was used for normally distributed data whereas the Kruskal Wallis followed by Dunn's test was applied for not normally distributed data. Sample size, specific tests and statistical details are given with the respective figures. Differences were considered significant if $p < 0.05$ (* $p<0.05$, ** $p<0.01$).

4 Results

4.1 Transfection of PMN with different doses of miRNA mimics

To test the transfection protocol and find an appropriate transfection concentration for the selected miRNA, PMN were transfected with final well concentrations of 0.5 nM, 5 nM or 50 nM double stranded syn-mmu-miR-132-3p respectively syn-mmu-miR-212-3p mimics. As a negative control, cells were transfected with 5 nM NC siRNA. RNA was isolated, transcribed to cDNA and miRNA levels were measured by qRT-PCR (Figure 3).

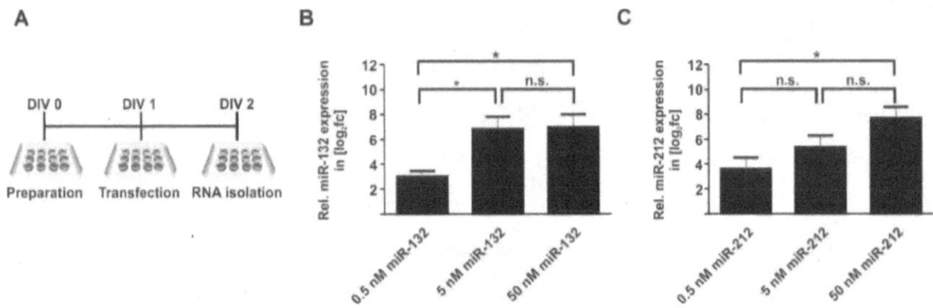

Figure 3 Transfection of PMN with miRNA mimics

(A) Experimental plan for testing transfection with different miRNA mimic concentrations. After transfection with different concentrations of miRNA mimics or NC at DIV 1, RNA was isolated at DIV 2 (24 h post-transfection). (B/C) Expression levels of miR-132-3p (B; experiment conducted by L. Caldi Gomes, (Caldi Gomes 2016)) and miR-212-3p (C) after transfection with synthetic miRNA mimics at 0.5 nM, 5 nM and 50 nM final well concentration. RNU6 expression was used as endogenous control. Data were analyzed with the ΔΔCT method and are shown as mean ± SEM expressed in $\log_2$ fold change (fc, both n = 4). Data were analyzed by one-way ANOVA followed by pair-wise comparison using Tukey's post-hoc test and are given as mean ± SEM. * $p < 0.05$

Figure 3 shows the miR-132-3p (B) and miR-212-3p (C) levels after transfection with the indicated concentrations of miRNA mimics relative to endogenous expression levels in NC transfected cells as analyzed by the ΔΔCT method. Both miRNAs show increased expression levels indicating that the miRNA mimics successfully transfected the cells. The miRNA levels measured by qRT-PCR also increased with increasing transfection concentrations showing a clear dose-dependent effect. The levels of miR-132-3p increased to 3.02 $\log_2$ fc for the 0.5 nM concentration and reached a plateau with an increase of 6.85 $\log_2$ fc for the 5 nM respectively 7.00 $\log_2$ fc for the 50 nM concentration. Both, the 5 nM and the 50 nM concentration of miR-132-3p mimics led to significantly higher levels in qPCR compared to the 0.5 nM condition.

For miR-212-3p expression increased to 3.60 log_2 fc for 0.5 nM, to 5.40 log_2 fc for 5 nM and to 7.70 log_2 fc for the 50 nM transfection concentration. Here, only the miRNA levels between the 0.5 nM and the 50 nM concentration of miR-212-3p mimics were significantly different. To compare the effects of the two miRNA mimics in the following experiments, 5 nM was selected as suitable transfection concentration.

4.2 Increased levels of miR-132-3p enhanced neurite growth in dopaminergic PMN

To evaluate the influence of increased levels of miRNA-132-3p and miRNA-212-3p in dopaminergic PMN, cells were plated on coverslips, transfected with 5 nM miRNA mimics at DIV 1 (Figure 4-A) and fixated for analysis at DIV 4. Staining against TH was used to exclusively label dopaminergic neurons and look for possible alterations in only this specific type of neurons. The total neurite length per TH positive cell was quantified relatively to the respective NC transfected cells of the same culture and is displayed in Figure 4-B.

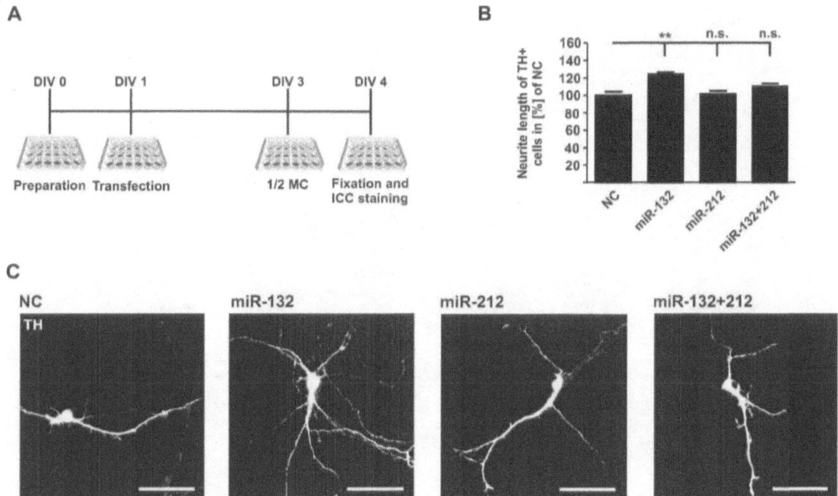

Figure 4 Elevated miR-132-3p levels increase neurite length in dopaminergic PMN

(A) Experimental scheme for the investigation of neurite length after transfection with 5 nM miRNA mimics at DIV 1 (1/2 MC = half of the wells' medium changed). (B) Quantification of the total neurite length per TH positive cell in different experimental conditions normalized to NC siRNA transfected cultures (miR-132 n = 6, miR-212 n = 10, miR-132+212 n = 9). (C) Representative micrographs of TH positive PMN of all experimental conditions as indicated (scale bar 50 μm). Data were analyzed by one-way ANOVA with Dunnett's post-hoc test and are given as mean ± SEM. ** $p<0.01$.

Transfection with 5 nM miR-132-3p mimics led to a significant increase of neurite outgrowth in dopaminergic PMN by 24.0 ± 2.0 % SEM ($p = 0.0034$). On the other hand, neither the transfection with miR-212-3p (101.4 ± 3.6 % SEM, $p = 0.98$) nor the combined transfection with both miRNAs (110.0 ± 1.1 % SEM, $p = 0.25$) altered neurite outgrowth (Figure 4-B). Interestingly, the combined transfection of both miRNAs diminished the beneficial effect of miR-132-3p on neurite outgrowth of dopaminergic PMN.

4.3 Elevated levels of miR-132-3p improve regeneration of dopaminergic neurites after scratch lesion

On DIV 1, PMN were transfected with 5 nM miRNA mimics or NC siRNA. Neurites were transected by a scratch lesion at DIV 2 (Figure 5-A). After fixation at DIV 4 and immunostaining against TH, the length of regenerating dopaminergic neurites crossing the scratch border was measured.

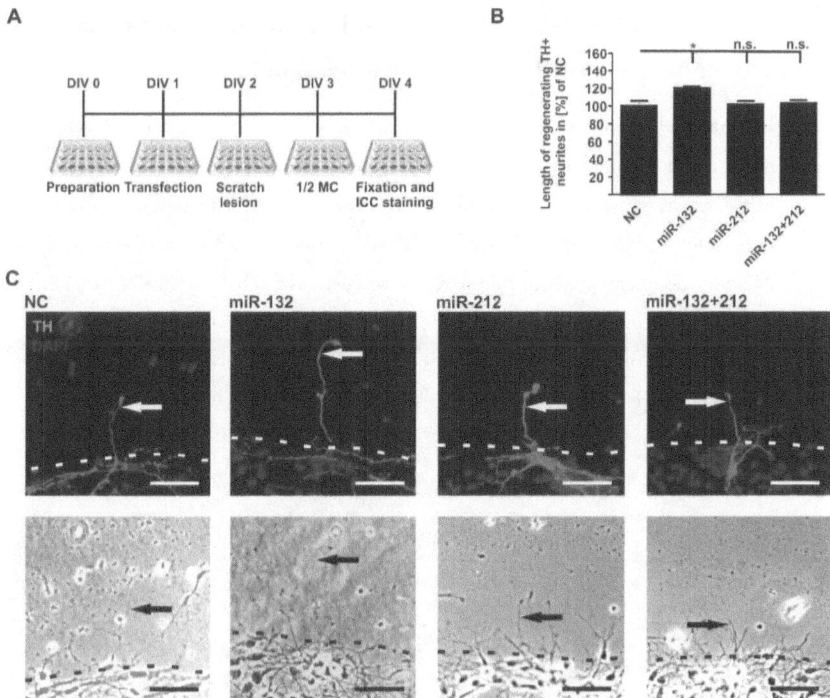

Figure 5 Only miR-132-3p improves regeneration after scratch lesion in dopaminergic PMN

(A) Experimental plan to investigate the neurite regeneration of TH positive neurons after scratch lesion. Cells were transfected at DIV 1, neurites transected at DIV 2 and fixated at DIV 4. (B) Relative neurite length of the seven longest neurites per image normalized to NC siRNA transfected PMN (miR-132 n = 5, miR-212 n = 9, miR-132+212 n = 10). (C) Exemplary brightfield (bottom) and fluorescent (TH immunostained and DAPI counter stained) (top) micrographs of transfected PMN with a dotted line indicating the scratch border (conditions as indicated; scale bar 50 μm). Data were analyzed by one-way ANOVA with Dunnett's test and are given as mean ± SEM. * $p < 0.05$

The results displayed in Figure 5 show that transfection with 5 nM miR-132-3p mimics significantly increases neurite regeneration by 20.0 % ± 1.8 % SEM compared to NC siRNA treated cells ($p = 0.046$, $n = 5$). Transfection with miR-212-3p (101.5 % ± 4.0 % SEM, $p = 0.9921$, $n = 9$) or miR-132-3p+212-3p (102.9 % ± 3.6 % SEM, $p = 0.95$, $n = 10$) did not alter neurite regeneration of TH positive neurons relative to NC siRNA transfected cultures (Figure 5-B).

4.4 Neither miR-132-3p nor miR-212-3p mimics have neuroprotective effects in MPP+ treated dopaminergic PMN

In order to investigate a possible beneficial effect of higher levels of miR-132-3p and miR-212-3p on the survival of dopaminergic neurons, the catecholaminergic neurotoxin MPP^+ was used which leads to specific degeneration of dopaminergic neurons. Cells were transfected with 5 nM miRNA mimics at DIV 1 and 2 μM MPP^+ were applied at DIV 2 for 24 hours. Supplemented cell culture media was used as a vehicle control. At DIV 3, the whole cell culture media was changed both for the treated and the vehicle control wells (Figure 6-A). After fixation at DIV4 and staining against TH, the number of TH positive somata was counted. The results are displayed in Figure 6.

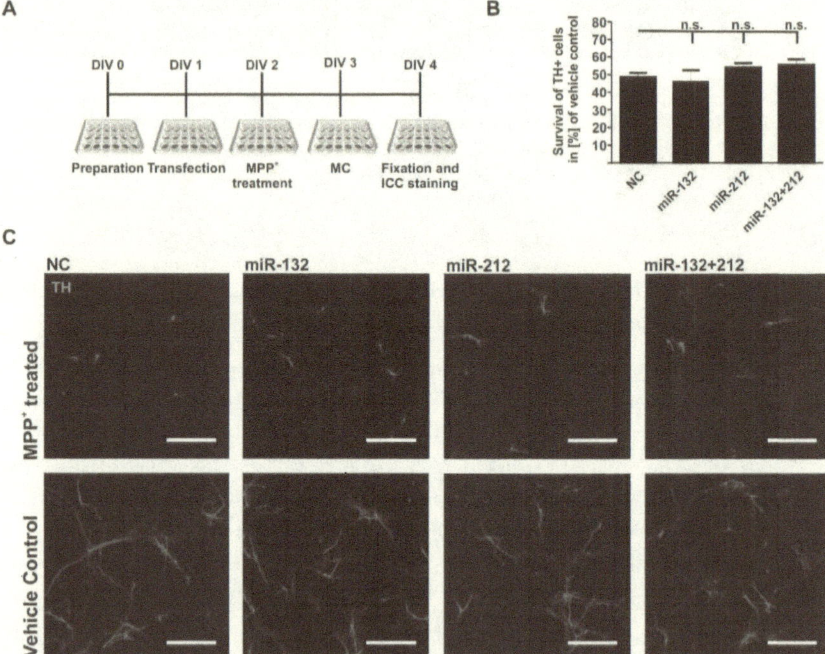

Figure 6 Survival of MPP^+ treated dopaminergic PMN is not altered by increased levels of miR-132-3p or miR-212-3p

(A) Experimental layout to investigate survival of TH positive neurons after 2 μM MPP^+ treatment. (B) Relative number of surviving TH positive cells in MPP^+ treated cultures, normalized to vehicle control (cell culture medium) treated PMN (miR-132-3p n = 3, miR-212-3p n = 6, miR-132-3p+212-3p n = 6). (C) Representative micrographs of TH immunostained MPP^+ treated (top row) and vehicle treated PMN (bottom row, scale bar 200 μm). Data were analyzed by one-way ANOVA with Dunnett's test and are given as mean ± SEM.

Treatment with 2 µM MPP^+ led to a stable decrease of TH positive neurons by ~50 % in all experimental conditions. Neither transfection with miR-132-3p nor with miR-212-3p mimics altered the survival of dopaminergic neurons after MPP^+ treatment. In NC siRNA treated wells, the number of TH positive cells was decreased to 48.6 % ± 0.7 % SEM (n = 10) compared to the cell culture medium treated vehicle control. For miR-132-3p transfected PMN, number of TH positive neurons was reduced to 45.7 % ± 3.9 % SEM (n = 3) and to 53.8 % ± 1.0 % SEM (n = 6) for miR-212-3p transfected PMN. The combined transfection of both miRNAs did not increase survival either (55.5 % ± 1.3 % SEM, Figure 6-B). Compared to NC siRNA transfected PMN the survival rate of TH positive neurons was not changed by none of the conditions.

4.5 miR-7b-5p and miR-129-2-3p do not alter neurite growth, neurite regeneration or survival of dopaminergic PMN

miR-7b-5p and miR-129-2-3p were also among the most regulated miRNA in the small RNA sequencing comparing the miRNAome of PMN at DIV 1 and DIV 5. Following the same hypothesis, that miRNA involved in maturation and growth could also act beneficial on dopaminergic neurons, the influence of increased miR-7b-5p and miR-129-2-3p levels was investigated under the same conditions as for the miR-132-3p and miR-212-3p (Figure 7).

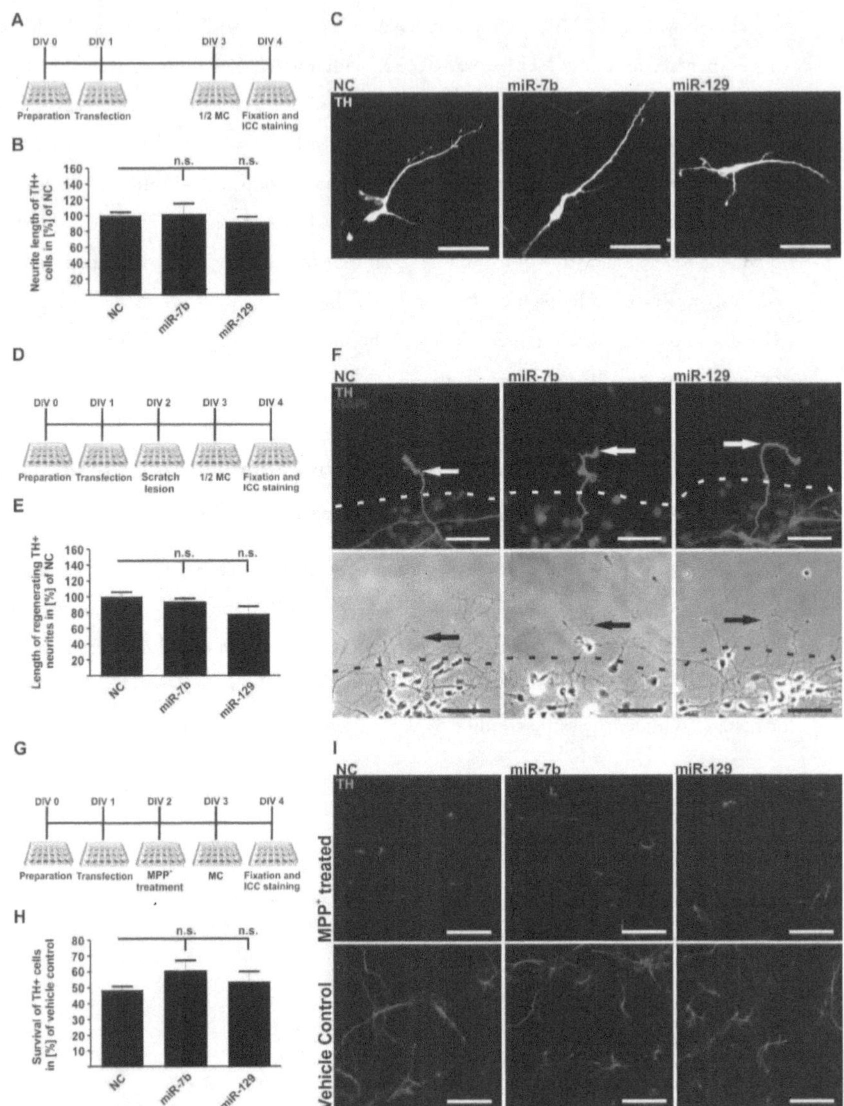

Figure 7 miR-7b-5p and miR-129-2-3p do not alter neurite growth, neurite regeneration after scratch lesion or survival of dopaminergic neurons after MPP^+ treatment in dopaminergic PMN

(A) Experimental layout for neurite growth analysis. (B) Relative neurite length per TH positive cell in miR-7b-5p and miR-129-2-3p transfected PMN normalized to NC siRNA treated cultures (both n = 4). (C) Representative micrographs of TH immunostained transfected PMN cultures (conditions as indicated; scale bar 50 µm).

[Legend of Figure 7] (D) Experiment layout to investigate neurite regeneration after scratch lesion. (E) Quantification of regenerating TH positive neurites after scratch lesion relative to NC (both n = 3). (F) Representative micrographs of TH immunostained and DAPI counter stained PMN with a dotted line indicating the scratch border (transfection conditions as indicated; scale bar 50 μm). (G) Experimental layout to investigate survival of dopaminergic PMN after treatment with 2 μM MPP+. (H) Quantification of surviving TH positive neurons after MPP+ treatment relative to vehicle treated control cultures (miR-7b-5p n = 6, miR-129-2-3p n = 5). (I) Representative micrographs of TH positive neurons treated with MPP+ (top row) or vehicle (bottom row; conditions as indicated; scale bar 200 μM). Data were analyzed by one-way ANOVA with Dunnett's test and are given as mean ± SEM.

Although the miR-7b-5p and miR-129-2-3p were also upregulated upon maturation, they did not alter neurite length of dopaminergic neurons. Dopaminergic PMN transfected with miR-7b-5p showed a neurite length of 100.6 % ± 14.7 % SEM (n = 4, p = 0.69) and miR-129-2-3p showed 90.1% ± 8.0 % SEM (n = 4, p = 0.33) compared to NC siRNA transfected cells (Figure 7 B). The two miRNAs did not alter regeneration of dopaminergic neurites after scratch lesion either. Compared to NC siRNA transfected PMN, the relative length of regenerating dopaminergic neurites was 93.9 % ± 4.0 % SEM (n = 3, p = 0.947) for miR-7b-5 and 78.5 % ± 9.7 % SEM (n = 3, p = 0.84) in miR-129-2-3p transfected dopaminergic PMN.

After treatment with 2 μM MPP+ the number of TH positive neurons in NC siRNA treated PMN was reduced to 48.6 % ± 0.7 % SEM (n = 10) compared with the vehicle control. In the miR-7b-5p transfected condition 56.4 % ± 2.3 % SEM (n = 6, p = 0.20) and 45.6 % ± 2.6 % SEM (n = 5, p = 0.72) of the miR129-2-3p transfected cells survived compared to the respective vehicle control. The two miRNAs did not show any neuro protective properties after MPP+ treatment either. The survival rate of none of the conditions was significantly different from NC siRNA transfected PMN (Figure 7 H).

4.6 LC/MS/MS proteome analysis of miR-132-3p and miR-212-3p transfected PMN

miRNA regulate gene expression by inhibition of mRNA translation and are thus affecting protein levels. In order to identify differentially regulated proteins after transfection with miR-132-3p or miR-212-3p mimics that might be relevant to the observed effects in the cell culture experiment, LC/MS/MS proteome analysis was employed. Cells were transfected with 5 nM miRNA mimics respectively NC siRNA at DIV 1 and lysed at DIV 3 (Figure 8-A). Three samples of 50 μg protein in a final volume of 30 μl were prepared from every culture.

A total of 4,349 proteins were identified at an FDR of 1 % by mapping the measured 623,867 MS/MS spectra to the UniProtKB *Mus musculus* reference proteome. After retention time correction to an iRT standard, 3,311 proteins could be quantified. The statistical analysis of differential protein expression was performed with the Significance B analysis of the Max Quant Perseus software (version 1.5.6.0).

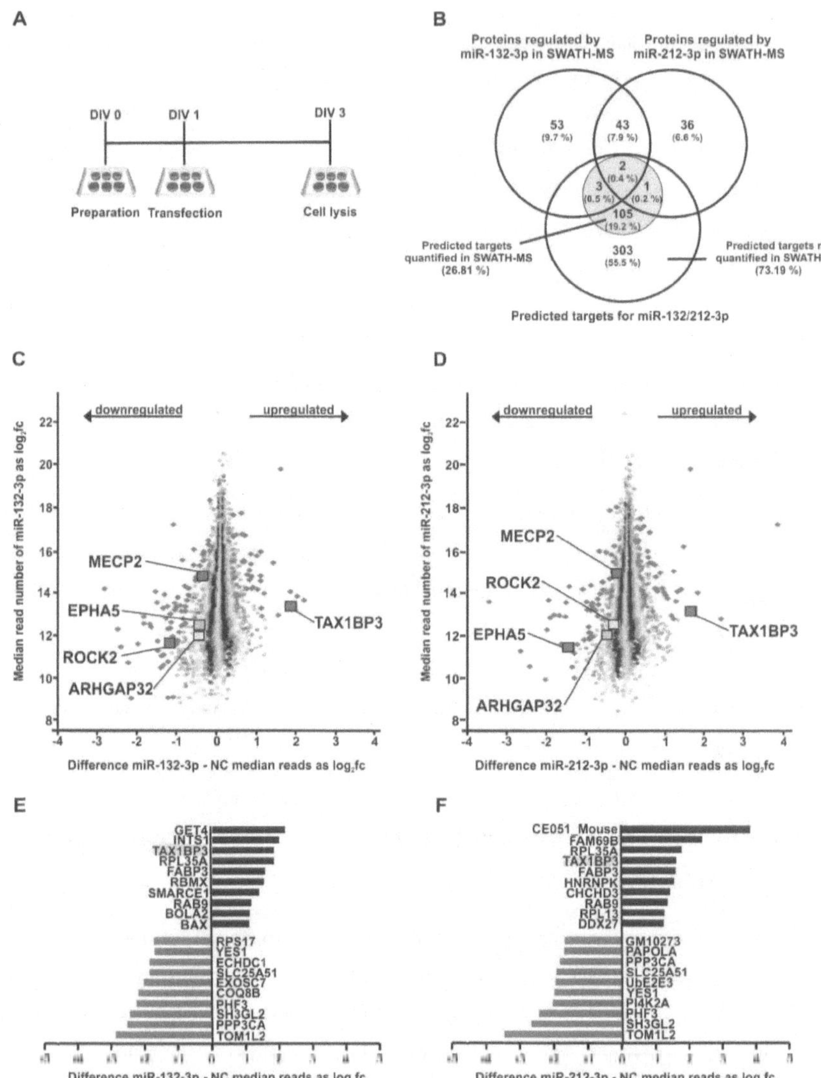

Figure 8 Proteome expression in miR-132-3p and miR-212-3p transfected PMN

[Legend of Figure 8] (A) Experimental layout for the investigation of protein expression using mass spectrometry. (B) The Venny diagram shows the overlap of differentially expressed proteins after transfection with miR-132-3p respectively miR-212-3p with predicted targets for their common seed sequence (targetscan.org). The part of the predicted targets also quantified in SWATH-MS is visualized as yellow circle within the lower circle of all predicted targets. The absolute numbers in an overlap of two or more circles means that this number of proteins matched to the criteria of more than one circle. In contrast, numbers enclosed by only one circle were found exclusively in the respective group. The total number of proteins in one group consist of the sum of all numbers enclosed by the respective circle. The percentages refer to the sum of all proteins from all four circles. (C/D) Differentially expressed proteins in SWATH-MS for miR-132-3p (C) and miR-212-3p (D) are depicted in a scatter plot. Less abundant proteins are found to the left, more abundant proteins to the right. The color of the dots reflects the significance according to the Significance B analysis of Perseus 1.5.6.0. Significantly different expressed proteins are displayed with larger diamonds in contrast to the smaller and not filled circles of not significantly regulated proteins. Proteins also investigated in Western Blot are named and highlighted. (E/F) The ten most up (blue) or down (red) regulated proteins for miR-132-3p (E) and miR-212-3p (F) are given as median log_2fc (n = 3). The protein TAX1BP3 is highlighted in red, as it was further evaluated in Western Blot.

In the miR-132-3p treated cells 101 proteins (3.1 % of all quantified proteins) were differentially expressed whereas only 83 proteins (2.5 %) were significantly altered in miR-212-3p transfected PMN compared to treatment with NC siRNA. Eleven proteins were similarly upregulated, and 24 proteins downregulated in both treatment conditions. This is an overlap in protein regulation of 38 % between the two miRNAs mimics transfected conditions. Opposite protein regulation with an upregulation in one and a downregulation in the other treatment condition was not observed. Out of 414 predicted targets only 111 (26.8 %) could be identified and quantified in the present SWATH-MS (yellow-circle in Figure 8-B).

The regulated proteins were mapped to the seed sequence-based target prediction by targetscan.org. The overlap of predicted targets and proteins regulated differentially in at least one condition in SWATH-MS is depicted in Figure 8-B and includes the following six proteins: PAPOLA and ARHGEF11 are the only proteins predicted for both and significantly downregulated by both miRNAs (overlap of all three circles). The overlap of predicted targets and proteins regulated in miR-132-3p transfected PMN included RRAS2, MECP2 and MAPT. While RRAS2 and MECP2 were downregulated, surprisingly, MAPT was upregulated. Since miRNA regulate gene expression by translational inhibition resulting in decreased protein expression, the upregulation of MAPT cannot be a direct effect of miR-132-3p but rather a downstream effect of the miRNA's targets. The same goes for the predicted target SRSF1 which was upregulated by miR-212-3p.

Other databases with different prediction algorithms identified 16 (microrna.org) or 67 (mirwalk.org) regulated proteins to be also predicted targets of miR-132-3p and 17 (microrna.org) or 65 (mirwalk.org) for miR-212-3p. An overview of proteins both regulated and predicted by the three different databases can be found in Table A2 in the appendix.

The significantly regulated proteins were imported to DAVID to identify involved KEGG pathways and GO clusters. DAVID revealed "Huntington's disease" (mmu05016), "Alzheimer's disease" (mmu05010) and "Tight junction" (mmu04530) to be significantly affected in the miR-132-3p transfected cells. The pathways and their regulated targets from SWATH-MS are displayed in Table 14. For miR-212-3p, no KEGG pathways were significantly involved.

Table 14 Significantly regulated KEGG pathways and corresponding differentially expressed proteins in SWATH-MS after transfection with miR-132-3p

Huntington's disease (mmu05016)	Alzheimer's disease (mmu05010)	Tight junction (mmu04530)
p = 3.23E-03	p = 9.57E-03	p = 1.90E-02
DLG4	HSD17B10	CSNK2B
NDUFA8	NDUFA8	RRAS2
NDUFS2	PPP3CA	GNAI1
BAX	MAPT	YES1
AP2M1	NDUFS2	TJP1
CASP3	CASP3	
DCTN2		

Furthermore, an analysis of the GO clusters of the differentially regulated proteins was performed with DAVID. The analysis revealed 13 regulated GO clusters for miR-132-3p and 7 for miR-212-3p mimic transfected PMN lysates and are displayed in Table A3 in the appendix.

Three significantly involved GO clusters of miR-132-3p targets and the respective proteins are given exemplary in Table 15. The GO clusters "Rho protein signal transduction" (GO:0007266), "Synapse assembly" (GO:0007416) and "Nervous system development" (GO:0007399) included among others MECP2 and ARHGEF11 which were already identified as predicted targets of miR-132-3p and miR-212-3p. Besides, these clusters are related to the growth-related questions addressed in the ICC experiments.

Table 15 Significantly involved GO cluster and corresponding differentially expressed proteins in SWATH-MS after transfection with miR-132-3p (three exemplary GO clusters)

Synapse assembly (GO:0007416)	Rho protein signal transduction (GO:0007266)	Nervous system development (GO:0007399)
p = 2.34E-02	p = 2.43E-02	p = 4.86E-02
GPM6A	ROCK2	CNTN1
SPTBN2	TAX1BP3	GPM6A
MECP2	ARHGEF11	SMARCE1
		CYFIP1
		NUMBL
		BAX

4.7 Analysis of protein expression in miR-132-3p and miR-212-3p treated PMN by Western blot

After the SWATH-MS proteomics already indicated several interesting proteins regulated by increased miR-132/212 levels and thus possibly relevant for the mediation of the observed neurobiological effects, the proteomics results had to be validated by another method. Besides already validated targets like MECP2 and ARHGAP32, three regulated proteins from SWATH-MS were selected exemplary for validation by Western blot – namely ROCK2, TAX1BP3 and EPHA5. These proteins were already reported earlier to be involved in regulation of neurite growth but not yet validated as targets of the miR-132/212 cluster. Out of these three proteins, levels of TAX1BP3 were increased in both conditions, whereas ROCK2 was exclusively downregulated in the miR-132-3p samples and EPHA5 only in miR-212-3p treated cells. The two proteins regulated exclusively in one condition were further investigated, to uncover underlying mechanism possibly explaining the different effects observed in ICC: To investigate the expression of the named proteins after transfection with one of the two miRNA mimics, PMN were transfected at DIV 1 and lysed at DIV 3 using RIPA buffer (Figure 9-A). Western blot analysis was performed with 25 µg protein per gel pocket. GAPDH was used as a housekeeping reference and protein levels are shown relative to levels in NC siRNA transfected cells.

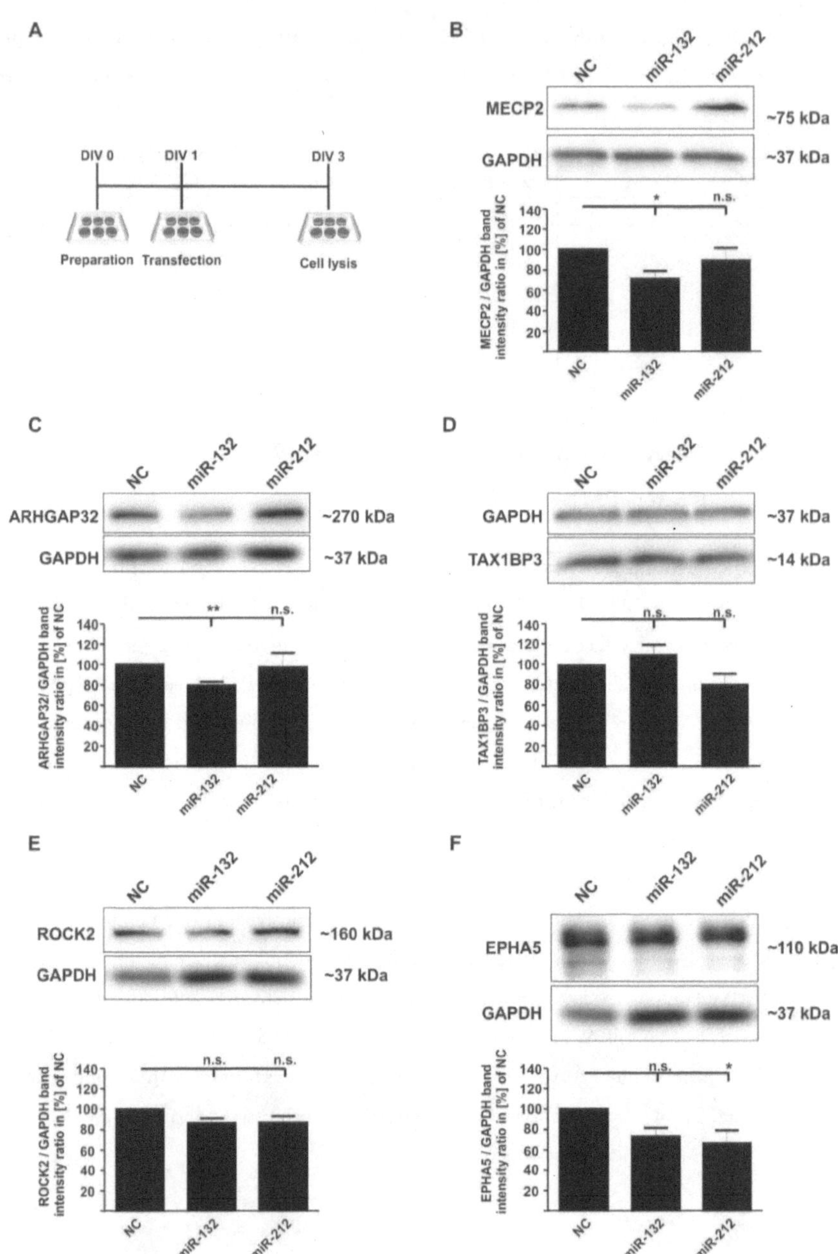

Figure 9 Expression of selected proteins of miR-132-3p or miR-212-3p transfected PMN in Western blot

(A) Experimental layout to investigate protein expression. (B-D) The Western blot analysis for (B) MECP2 (n = 10), (C) ARHGAP32 (n = 10), (D) TAX1BP3 (n = 9), (E) ROCK2 (n = 12) and (F) EPHA5 (n = 10).

[Legend of Figure 9] Data were first normalized to the loading control GAPDH and subsequently to the NC of the respective culture. Exemplary blot images of the loading control and the respective protein are shown below the graphs. Data were analyzed by one-way ANOVA with Dunnett's test and are given as mean ± SEM, with exception of ARHGAP32. For this protein data were not distributed normaly (Shapiro -Wilk Test p = 0.027) and were analyzed by the Kruskal Wallis and Dunn's test. * $p<0.05$, ** $p< 0.01$.

MECP2 is a predicted and validated target of both miRNAs and is also described to be involved in neuronal plasticity and morphogenesis. Indeed, its downregulation is reported to increase neurite length (Klein et al. 2007; Wada et al. 2010; Alvarez-Saavedra et al. 2011; Im et al. 2010; Bhattacherjee et al. 2017). In Western blot, MECP2 was found downregulated to 71.2 % ± 7.8 % SEM (p = 0.045) for miR-132-3p but not changed significantly for miR-212-3p (89.1 % ± 12.6 % SEM (p = 0.57 both n = 10, Dunnett's test, Figure 9-B). In SWATH MS, it was also only found downregulated for miR-132-3p (-0.38 median $\log_2$ fc).

The ARHGAP32 protein is also known under the no longer recommend term p250GAP. It was already shown to be regulated by miR-132-3p and to mediate neurite growth in other models (Vo et al. 2005; Magill et al. 2010). However, it was not expressed significantly different in the proteomics experiment (miR-132-3p: -0.47 median $\log_2$ fc). In Western blot, miR-132-3p transfected PMN had 20.7 % ± 3.4 % SEM (p = 0.001) decreased expression of ARHGAP32 whereas protein expression was not changed for miR-212-3p transfected PMN (97.2 % ± 14.1 %, p = 0.632, both n = 12, Kruskal Wallis and Dunn's test, Figure 9-C).

TAX1BP3 was significantly upregulated in SWATH-MS for both miRNAs (miR-132-3p: 1.85 median $\log_2$fc, miR-212-3p: 1.61 median $\log_2$fc). Surprisingly, the protein expression in Western blot was not significantly changed for none of the experimental conditions. The protein expression compared to NC siRNA treated cell was 110.0 % ± 9.2 % SEM (p=0.574) in miR-132-3p and 80.6 % ± 9.9 % SEM in miR-212-3p treated PMN (p=0.16, both n=9, Dunnett's test, Figure 9-D). According to mirwalk.org it is a predicted target of miR-212-3p but none of the target prediction algorithms lists TAX1BP3 as a target of miR-132-3p.

ROCK2 is a protein which is highly investigated in the context of ND but only mirwalk.org lists ROCK2 as a predicted target of miR-132-3p but not of miR-212-3p. Its downregulation leads to improved neurite growth and is probably beneficial in different ND (Koch et al. 2014; Koch et al. 2018). In mass spectrometry it was significantly downregulated for miR-132-3p (-1.19 median log_2 fc) but not changed for miR-212-3p. Western blot showed a trend to downregulation for both miRNAs not reaching statistical significance. The protein expression in miR-132-3p transfected cells was 86.4 % ± 4.7 % SEM ($p = 0.088$) and 86.7 % ± 6.7 % SEM ($p = 0.095$, both $n = 12$, Dunnett's test, Figure 9-E).

EPHA5 is a predicted target of miR-212-3p according to microrna.org and mirwalk.org and was significantly downregulated for miR-212-3p in SWATH-MS (-1.47 median log_2 fc). In Western blot it was significantly decreased to 66.4 % ± 12.8 % SEM ($p = 0.02$) in miR-212-3p transfected PMN compared to NC siRNA treatment. However, it also showed a similar trend in miR-132-3p transfected cells with a decrease to 73.1 % ± 8.6 % SEM not reaching statistical significance ($p = 0.08$, both $n = 9$, Dunnett's test, Figure 9-F).

5 Discussion

5.1 Modelling miRNA overexpression in PMN

This study intended to investigate effects of increased levels of the miR-132-3p and miR-212-3p in dopaminergic PMN. As the general efficacy of the PMN transfection protocol was already demonstrated earlier (Roser et al. 2018b), experiments to identify a suitable transfection concentration were performed with three different concentrations of the respective miRNA mimics. Transfection with 5 nM was identified as a suitable transfection concentration as no toxicity or saturation effect was observed. It was therefore used for both miRNAs in all following experiments.

The ICC and Western blot experiments showed that both miRNA mimics were transfected successfully and showed biological effects. The ICC and Western blot experiments revealed various effects of miR-132-3p in dopaminergic PMN, whereas the downregulation of EPHA5 was the only observed effect after transfection with miR-212-3p mimics. Based on the miRNA levels in qPCR, protein regulation and effects observed in ICC, one can conclude that the transfection with miRNA mimics is an appropriate *in vitro* model for the investigation of miRNA mediated effects and the involved protein alterations.

5.2 Possible mechanisms of increased neurite growth in miR-132-3p mimics treated dopaminergic PMN

Evaluating growth and regeneration of neuronal processes is highly relevant in the field of neurodegeneration. In PD, evidence suggests that the first neuropathological events start in the dopaminergic axons (Burke and O'Malley 2013). Our results have shown that miR-132-3p transfected PMN presented significant increase in neurite length and improved neurite regeneration after scratch lesion. Regulation of neurite morphogenesis and arborization by miR-132-3p was already demonstrated in cortical, newborn olfactory bulb and hippocampal neurons (Vo et al. 2005; Pathania et al. 2012; Magill et al. 2010; Impey et al. 2010). Interestingly, these studies either used a knockout model of the whole miR-132/212 locus or exclusively investigated effects of increased levels of miR-132-3p. The neurite growth improving effect was attributed to the downregulation of ARHGAP32, which is a predicted target of miR-132-3p and was validated as a target in the context of the cited studies. Downregulation of ARHGAP32 activates the Rac-1-Pak signaling pathway leading to actin remodeling and neurite growth (Vo et al. 2005; Impey et al. 2010; Wayman et al.

2008). Here, we could confirm a downregulation of ARHGAP32 by miR-132-3p but not by miR-212-3p mimics in dopaminergic PMN by Western blot.

Further studies investigated the influence of miR-132-3p and novel mechanisms were identified to be involved in the mediation of its effects on axon growth. In dorsal root ganglia (DRG) miR-132-3p was shown to extend axon outgrowth via downregulation of RASA1 (also known as p120-RasGAP) in cell cultures locally in the axon (Hancock et al. 2014). Another putative mediator of neurite growth and especially neurite arborization is MECP2. It was found downregulated for miR-132-3p in SWATH-MS and Western blot whereas levels for miR-212-3p were not changed. Moreover, our SWATH-MS experiments identified the significantly regulated GO cluster "*Synapse assembly*" including MECP2 together with GPM6A and SPTBN2 (Table 15). The MECP2 protein is an already validated target both for miR-132-3p and miR-212-3p (Klein et al. 2007; Wada et al. 2010; Im et al. 2010). A knockout of *Mecp2* was demonstrated to lead to improved neurite growth in *Mecp2* deficient DRG. The downregulation of MECP2 by miR-132-3p could thus be co-responsible for the enhanced neurite growth induced by miR-132-3p (Bhattacherjee et al. 2017). However, the effects of MECP2 in regulating neurite growth are complex and might be affected by several regulatory mechanisms. There is considerable evidence that both – decreased as well as increased levels – impair cognition and development. For instance, mutation in the MECP2 locus lead to the X-linked Rett's syndrome including massive cognitive deficits. It is also reported to be involved in a homeostatic control of BDNF, CREB and miR-132/212 transcription which all themselves regulate each other. For instance, miR-132-3p and miR-212-3p are reported to indirectly suppress BDNF expression but also to initiate a BDNF disinhibition by targeting the BDNF inhibitor MECP2 (Im et al. 2010). Thereby the miRNAs contribute to the homeostasis of BDNF. The expression of CREB is stimulated among others also via a disinhibition mediated by miRNA induced downregulation of MECP2. Both, the transcription factor CREB and the neurotrophic BDNF, are highly important for neurodevelopment and neuronal plasticity – processes where a correct function of miR-132/212 is also needed. The direct miRNA target MECP2 but also CREB and BDNF are likely to be parts of the miR-132/212 influenced mechanisms upon the mentioned processes (Feng and Nestler 2010; Im et al. 2010). Additionally, both CREB and BDNF, control the transcription of miR-132/212 (Vo et al. 2005; Remenyi et al. 2010).

Another significantly regulated GO cluster from our SWATH-MS results, features the biological process *"Rho protein signal transduction"*. It includes ROCK2, TAX1BP3 and ARHGEF11. Inhibition of ROCK2 has already been described to improve neurite outgrowth (Lingor et al. 2007; Fuentes et al. 2008; Koch et al. 2014).

The ROCK2 protein was also found downregulated in our analysis as shown by SWATH-MS after miR-132-3p transfection and showed a similar trend after transfection of both miRNAs in Western blot validation studies. This downregulation could be an additional mediator of improved neurite outgrowth induced by miR-132-3p. Experiments in zebrafish nerve explants also demonstrated an involvement of TAX1BP3 in neurite outgrowth. Its siRNA-mediated downregulation led to shorter neurites, but this effect could be rescued by an additional inhibition of ROCK (Matsukawa et al. 2018). Although TAX1BP3 was highly upregulated in SWATH-MS for both conditions, no alterations of protein expression could be observed in Western blot.

Furthermore, the growth-related protein MAPT (also known as TAU) was upregulated in our SWATH-MS results for miR-132-3p transfected PMN but is also a predicted target of both miRNA strands. The miR-132-3p is even validated to target MAPT and its deficiency is reported to decrease neurite growth in embryonic hippocampal neurons (Dawson et al. 2001). Thus, the upregulation of MAPT in miR-132-3p transfected PMN is compatible with the growth improving effects observed in miR-132-3p treated cultures. On the other hand, the validation of MAPT as a target of miR-132-3p in miR-132/212 deficient mice and neuroblastoma cells transfected with miR-132-3p mimics is contradictory to the SWATH-MS results. After transfection with miR-132-3p one would expect a downregulation of MAPT, however, it was upregulated in the SWATH-MS analysis for the miR-132-3p condition. As both – high levels of miR-132-3p and of MAPT– are associated with improved growth upon maturation, a context-dependent regulation of MAPT by miR-132-3p is possible. Whereas MAPT may be downregulated by miR-132-3p in mature neurons, it is possibly not directly targeted by miR-132-3p in maturing neurons such as the PMN used here. Thus, further analysis of MAPT regulation by miR-132/212 in maturing neurons is needed. Moreover, the protein is intensively investigated because its aggregation in mature neurons was demonstrated to lead to different kinds of ND such as AD and different types of aPS; the so called tauopathies. (Smith et al. 2015; Zuo et al. 2016; Dawson et al. 2001; Coppede 2012).

The experiments presented here showed a downregulation of ARHGAP32 and MECP2 by miR-132-3p and the same trend was observed for ROCK2. Downregulation of these proteins was repeatedly reported to increase neurite growth and could thus be partly responsible for the growth improving effects of miR-132-3p on dopaminergic PMN observed in ICC experiments. However, to attribute the growth improving effects directly to these proteins, further experiments specifically targeting these proteins (e.g. via siRNA) are necessary.

5.3 miR-132-3p induced improvement of neurite regeneration in dopaminergic PMN and possible underlying mechanisms

The scratch lesion experiments were performed to further elucidate regeneration abilities of dopaminergic neurons with increased levels of miR-132-3p and miR-212-3p. Our results indicate that transfection with miR-132-3p mimics – but not with miR-212-3p mimics – led to improved regeneration after scratch lesion (measured as sum of the seven longest neurites normalized to the NC). Thus, this observation could possibly be influenced by neurite growth pathways, in case that neurite growth and neurite regeneration base on common on similar pathways and mechanisms. However, experiments with cultured neurons of Drosophila revealed that major pathways like PI3K/Akt and TOR were necessary for neurite regeneration and sprouting, but not for the initial neurite growth (Marmor-Kollet and Schuldiner 2016). Another study in cultures of cortical neuron described morphological differences and a different cytoskeletal composition of growth cones of growing and regenerating neurons (Blizzard et al. 2007). They also reported that GDNF and BDNF enhanced growth of developing but not of regenerating axons indicating the existence of different underlying pathways. However, another study observed improved regeneration after scratch lesion in GDNF transfected dopaminergic neurons (Roser et al. 2018b). The same scratch lesion model in dopaminergic PMN was also used by Saal and colleagues (2015) who observed a massively improved neurite regeneration after inhibition of ROCK2 by short-hairpin-RNA (shRNA) expressing AAV. As ROCK2 was also downregulated after miR-132-3p transfection shown by SWATH-MS and showed a similar trend in the Western blot validation, ROCK2 might be one of the mediators of improved neurite regeneration in the present model.

Earlier studies which showed an enhanced regeneration after scratch lesion also investigated possible underlying cellular mechanisms. It was observed that the applied regeneration improving treatments involved TGF-β-modulated proteasome activity, JNK activity, downregulation of the pro-autophagic FOXO3 and activation of the pro survival PI3K-Akt signaling pathway (Tonges et al. 2011; Knöferle et al. 2010; Roser et al. 2018b). These findings suggest that the observed regeneration after mechanical lesion is at least partly mediated by modulation of apoptosis and autophagy. Interestingly, FOXO3 is also a validated target of miR-132-3p and miR-212-3p (Byeon et al. 2017; Mehta et al. 2015). Also the activation of the PI3K-Akt signaling pathway was described via a miR-132-3p induced downregulation of PTEN in a human brain endothelial cell line and primary cortical neurons (Gu et al. 2018; Zhao et al. 2018).

Taken together, the present literature suggests different targets and pathways influenced by increased levels miR-132-3p related to apoptosis and autophagy which could also be partly responsible for the effects observed here. To test putative underlying pathways or proteins, similar experiments specifically regulating single proteins (e.g. by siRNA) are needed. Western blot and SWATH-MS indicated first promising candidates such as ROCK2 or PTEN.

5.4 Transfection with miR-132-3p or miR-212-3p mimics cannot protect dopaminergic neurons from MPP$^+$ induced toxicity

Research strives to provide neuroprotective therapies to PD patients who are currently only treated symptomatically. An optimal disease-modifying therapy would slow down the progression of the degenerative processes. Toxicity induced by MPP$^+$ specifically targets dopaminergic neurons which are the predominantly affected cell type in PD. It leads to massive oxidative stress by complex I inhibition which is also suspected to play a role in PD pathogenesis (Kopin 1992; Dexter and Jenner 2013; Puspita et al. 2017). In the present experiments, none of the miRNA mimics transfected conditions improved the survival of the dopaminergic neurons. In earlier studies, inhibition of ROCK2 by transduction with shRNA expressing AAV was shown to improve survival of dopaminergic neurons after MPP$^+$ treatment (Saal et al. 2015). They thereby applied a much more specific treatment targeting a single protein than we achieved by the transfection with miRNA targeting an incalculable number of targets. The possible miRNA mimics induced downregulation of ROCK2 might be insufficient to significantly influence neuronal survival after MPP$^+$ treatment. Furthermore, the influence of other pathways on neuronal survival affected by the miRNA treatment cannot be estimated.

Another mechanisms of improved neuronal survival are the earlier discussed downregulation of FOXO3 or activation of the PI3K-pathway described in a similar experiment with PMN (Roser et al. 2018b). Among the discussed targets, ROCK2 is the only one detected in the SWATH-MS analysis where it was downregulated in miR-132-3p transfected PMN with a similar trend in Western blot. Other proteins like the PI3K pathway controlling PTEN or FOXO3 were neither detected in SWATH-MS nor were they investigated in Western blot here. Thus, it is unclear whether they are regulated as suggested in the present model. Besides, our results might indicate an insufficient regulation of the relevant pathways in relation to the applied toxin. Nevertheless, earlier studies in PMN with miR-182-5p and miR-183-5p treated with the same concentrations of MPP$^+$ and miRNA mimics, however, did observe beneficial effects in miRNA transfected PMN (Roser et al. 2018b). The applied MPP^+ dosage of 2 µM is therefore probably not generally excessively toxic but leaves leeway for possible miRNA mediated neuroprotective effects as observed by Roser and colleagues. Consequently, the effects of the treatment with miRNA mimics used in the present study might be not specific enough or insufficient in their regulation of ROCK2 or other not investigated mechanisms to induce any observable effects against the dopaminergic neurotoxicity induced by MPP^+.

Other reports described effects of another miRNA from the miR-132/212 cluster. Sun and colleagues published a comprehensive study on the effects of the counter strand miR-212-5p, which they observed to be downregulated both in MPTP *in vivo* and MPP^+ *in vitro* models. Injection of miR-212-5p mimics into the lateral ventricle was shown to protect dopaminergic neurons from MPTP induced cell death. Survival of dopaminergic neurons was also improved in MPP^+ treated SH-SY5Y cells with increased levels of mR-212-5p. They attributed the observed effect to the downregulation of the cytosolic SIRT2 which was upregulated after MPTP and MPP^+ treatment but downregulated by the miR-212-5p mimics. The neuroprotective effect was probably mediated by consecutive downregulation of p53 (Sun et al. 2018). Earlier studies also demonstrated neuroprotective effects of SIRT2 inhibitors (Outeiro et al. 2007). In the SWATH-MS analysis the expression of SIRT2 was not altered for none of the miRNA neither is it a predicted target of the miR-132-3p or miR-212-3p strands used in this study. However, it is interesting to notice that the 5p-counter strands have neuroprotective effects as they are transcribed as common pri-miRNA even though the 3p strands are reported to be the predominantly processed miRNAs.

The experiment with MPP^+ induced cell toxicity was also conducted with PMN transfected with other miRNA – namely the miR-7b-5p and miR-129-2-3p – previously identified as putative players in dopaminergic development *in vitro* (Roser 2016). In our experiments, the aforementioned miRNAs did not alter survival of dopaminergic neurons either. Other studies however, did observe attenuated cell death for miR-7b-5p in SH-SY5Y cells (Li et al. 2016) and in cortical neurons transduced with miR-7b carrying AAV (Choi et al. 2014). Li and colleagues also attributed the attenuated cell death to the downregulation of SIRT2 and BAX which they found downregulated in Western blot. As miR-7b-5p also targets α-synuclein, it has been discussed as a potential therapeutic agent in PD (Titze-de-Almeida and Titze-de-Almeida 2018). For miR-129 and miR-132, there are no comparable studies available.

Although the mentioned studies investigating effects of miR-7b or miR-212-5p are partially related to the experiments presented here, they were fundamentally different in several important aspects. Sun and colleagues used the counter strand of the miR-212-3p that was used here. The studies on miR-7b used different models, different miRNA vehicles or did not focus exclusively on dopaminergic neurons. Nevertheless, the reported effects of miR-212-5p or miR-7b-5p make these miRNAs promising therapeutic agents against MPP^+ induced dopaminergic degeneration.

5.5 SWATH-MS and target validation in Western blot

The SWATH-MS analysis served as a discovery method for altered protein abundancies related to treatment with miRNA mimics in PMN. In this context, it is important to highlight that miRNA regulate protein levels by binding to the respective mRNA before translation or further post translational modifications take place (Winter et al. 2009; Wang et al. 2013b). Changes induced by miRNA mimics can therefore be hidden by compensatory effects such as a slower degradation of the respective proteins. Furthermore, the measured differences between the experimental conditions can be the result of direct effects of the transfected miRNA mimics but can also due to a reactive counter regulation or downstream effects of affected pathways. Finally, by quantitative protein measurement, it is not possible to make any statements on the function of proteins, i.e. activities of kinases and other enzymes.

The present SWATH-MS results revealed an interesting overlap of miRNA predicted targets and regulated proteins. Out of 3,311 quantified proteins 101 (3.1 %) were regulated by miR-132-3p and 83 (2.5 %) by miR-212-3p. Targetscan.org predicts 414 targets for the mmu-miR-for these miRNAs. Out of these 414 predicted targets, 111 could be detected and quantified in our experiments. From those, six proteins that are also predicted targets of the miR-132/212 cluster were indeed regulated. Finally, four targets were at the same time predicted and downregulated – as expected in the canonical miRNA regulation of the transcriptome and the potential modulation in protein expression. Those were PAPOLA and ARHGEF11 (downregulated by both miRNAs), as well as RRAS2 and MECP2 (only regulated by miR-132-3p).

The limited overlap of predicted targets and quantified proteins might be because the used cell lysates from PMN only include two different cell types – GABAergic (90-95 %) and dopaminergic neurons (5-10 %). They do thus not include all possible proteins. Furthermore, the number of quantified proteins was reduced technically as only proteins identified in every run and sample were considered for quantification. Moreover, data independent acquisition methods such as SWATH-MS reveal predominantly differences of the most abundant proteins. Less abundant proteins – which are probably more expressed in non-neuronal tissue or more mature cells – may not have been expressed sufficiently to be quantified. Other methods of mass spectrometry analysis concentrating on lists of predefined targets like *peptide centric scoring* (also called *targeted data extraction*) can be three- to ten-fold more sensitive than SWATH-MS and would thus be more suitable to investigate less abundant proteins and peptides (Ludwig et al. 2018).

It is important to mention that the target prediction databases employed here are mainly based on matching sequences of the miRNAs' seed regions to those of mRNAs, and thus, still include many false-positive and non-validated proteins. During the statistical analysis of SWATH-MS data, it was also noticed that the three different PMN cultures differed quite substantially from each other. Therefore, it is likely that several regulated proteins did not reach statistical significance as the variability between the different cell cultures was too high. On the other hand, our SWATH-MS experiments detected MECP2, a predicted and repeatedly validated target of miR-132-3p (Im et al. 2010; Wada et al. 2010; Klein et al. 2007). Besides, there are no comparable studies published to estimate the quality and results of this SWATH-MS. A recent proteome analysis of the nucleus suprachiasmaticus from miR-132/212 deficient mice analyzed the time-of-day dependent fluctuation in the knockout proteome. They identified among others *Ephrin Receptor Signaling*, *RhoGDI signaling* and *Remodeling of epithelial tight junctions* as time-of-day dependent GO clusters in the miR-132/212 knockout mice, which fits to KEGG pathways and targets discussed in the context of the present SWATH-MS analysis (Mendoza-Viveros et al. 2017).

An interesting study in this context investigated the hippocampal mRNA expression of miR-132/212 deficient, miR-132 and miR-212 overexpressing mice. They only considered mRNAs as targets which were downregulated in the overexpressing animals, upregulated in the knockout mice and predicted by microRNA.org. This resulted in 13 targets regulated by miR-132 and one target regulated by miR-212. Five of the miR-132 regulated targets were also detected in the present SWATH-MS analysis but none of them was regulated significantly. The only protein fulfilling all three criteria for miR-212 was STX1A which was not detected in the present SWATH-MS (Hansen et al. 2016).

Mass spectrometry proteomics with SWATH analysis can record treatment induced protein alterations on a large scale and unbiased for the selection of proteins. However, it quantifies protein expression without a loading control to normalize for varying loading amounts. Therefore, single proteins related to neurite growth and regeneration were selected for validation by Western blot where protein expression can be normalized to a loading control, such as GAPDH which is not altered by the applied treatment. The experimental protocol of transfecting the PMN with the miRNA mimics until the lysis of the cells using RIPA buffer and a sonication device, was the same for the SWATH-MS and the Western blot samples. In the cases of MECP2 and EPHA5, results from SWATH-MS could be validated successfully by Western blot. MECP2 was downregulated by miR-132-3p in both experiments and EPHA5 was downregulated for miR-212-3p in both cases.

ROCK2 was significantly decreased after miR-132-3p transfection in SWATH-MS. In Western blot it showed a similar trend for both miRNAs, yet no significant regulation. In this context, it is important to underline that effects of kinases like ROCK2 depend more on their activity than on their absolute quantity. Its activity can be regulated, for instance, by deletion of the auto-inhibiting carboxyl-terminal region (constitutive activation), binding of RHOA for (transient disinhibition) and phosphorylation (Koch et al. 2018). This means that the physiological effects of ROCK2 must be additionally assessed by measuring its activity and by measuring the modulation of its downstream targets.

Besides, TAX1BP3 – which was reported to be necessary for neurite outgrowth (Matsukawa et al. 2018) – was selected for validation. In SWATH-MS, it was highly upregulated and was among the ten most upregulated proteins in both conditions. This effect could not be reproduced in Western blot, where no significant differences were observed. For miR-212-3p there was even a mild (non-significant) trend towards decreased TAX1BP3 expression. Since Western blot is a technique widely used to validate proteomics results – despite of its technical limitations – the TAX1BP3 results obtained by Western blot with ten independent PMN cultures are more credible than the proteomics results. Interestingly, TAX1BP3 is a predicted target of miR-212-3p, but not of miR-132-3p.

All in all, our Western blot analyses could confirm the regulation of most of the selected proteins. Nevertheless, the SWATH-MS results revealed more targets than analyzed and discussed here. Because of limitations in time and scope, we reduced our selection of validated proteins to those directly related to neurite growth and regeneration.

5.6 Possible mechanisms and pathways mediating the effects observed in ICC

In order to link regulated targets and related pathways of miR-132-3p and miR-212-3p to each other and to the neurite growth and neurite regeneration improving effects observed in ICC, observations from SWATH-MS and Western blots were compiled alongside with an extensive literature research. Therefore, reports mentioning miR-132-3p and miR-212-3p in the context of neurite growth, regeneration and maturation as well as three different target prediction databases were considered. The proposed protein interactions and pathways are displayed in Figure 10. The results from the named experiments and specific references from literature research for all discussed targets are summarized in the appendix in Table A4.

The complex effects of altered MECP2 levels and the feedback loop controlling miR-132/212 transcription were discussed earlier and are not implemented in the figure. TAX1BP3 is not included in the figure as its results from SWATH-MS and Western blot were contradictory. Moreover, this protein and its interactions are still poorly understood. So far, it was only reported that TAX1BP3 is necessary for neurite growth in zebrafish nerve explants. It possibly increases neurite growth by inactivation of RHOA via rhotekin (RTKN). Besides, impaired neurite growth after TAX1BP3 siRNA treatment can be rescued by ROCK inhibition (Matsukawa et al. 2018). Regulation of cell development via MAPT was also not implemented due to the contradictions discussed.

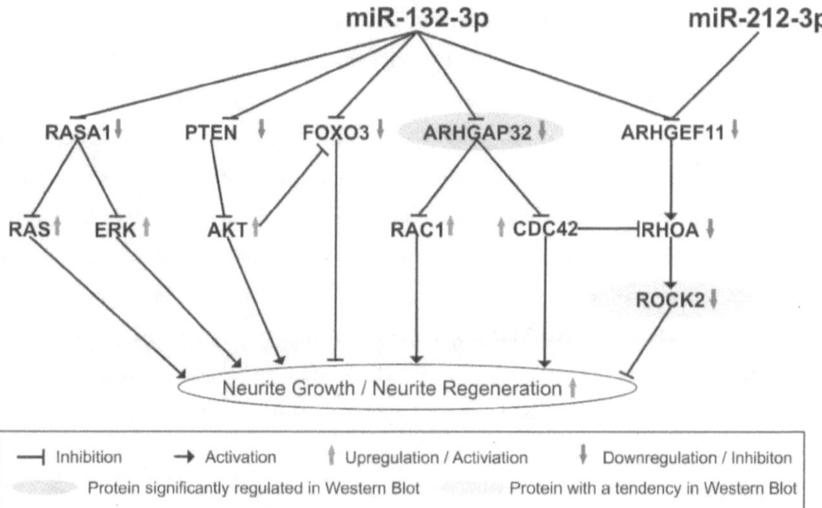

Figure 10 Proposed proteins and pathways altered by overexpression of miR-132-3p and miR-212-3p possibly mediating the effects observed in ICC experiments

Targets of miR-132-3p and miR-212-3p validated in this book or other publications are summarized and linked to their influence on neurite growth and neurite regeneration. The green or red arrows indicate the respective protein regulation after increased levels of miR-132-3p and miR-212-3p. Proteins investigated in the present study are highlighted in yellow. This simplified figure does not differentiate between influences on neurite growth and neurite regeneration as many of the pathways were described to be involved both in neurite growth and regeneration. Table A4 summarizes experimental results, target prediction and results from other publications for all targets shown in this figure.

According to the pathways depicted here, by targeting PTEN, miR-132-3p induces a disinhibition of the PI3K signaling pathway and a consequently upregulation of its targets like CREB, mTOR or AKT. The pathway is especially important for the regulation of the cell cycle and cell proliferation. It is considered as a major pro-survival pathway – alterations were therefore also frequently observed in cancer studies (Gu et al. 2018; Wong et al. 2013; Liu et al. 2017; Jin et al. 2012). Nevertheless, inhibition of PTEN was demonstrated to induce neurite growth and, in particular, to enhance neurite regeneration. In this context, a therapeutic inhibition of PTEN in CNS disorders and after axonal injury is also discussed (Ohtake et al. 2015; Park et al. 2008). On the other hand, experiments with Drosophila mushroom body neurons revealed that PI3K/Akt and TOR were necessary for neurite regeneration and sprouting, but not for the initial neurite growth (Marmor-Kollet and Schuldiner 2016).

The transcription factor FOXO3 can be inhibited by the PI3K downstream target AKT but is also a direct target of both miR-132-3p and miR-212-3p. As it has pro-apoptotic effects, its downregulation is linked to improved neuronal survival and neurite regeneration, but also to carcinogenesis (Roser et al. 2018b; Santo et al. 2013; Wong et al. 2013; Mehta et al. 2015; Wang et al. 2013a). The miR-132-3p induced anti-apoptotic effects of increased PI3K and decreased FOXO3 activity were even used to explain the increased apoptosis in AD. In a study using brain tissue of AD patients, the levels of miR-132-3p and miR-212-3p were observed to be decreased depending on the disease state whereas the pro-apoptotic levels of PTEN, PI3K and FOXO3 increased. The direct influence of miR-132/212 on these targets was confirmed in different neuronal cell cultures and finally used as possible causal explanation for the increased neuronal apoptosis observed in AD (Wong et al. 2013). An involvement of these apoptosis and cell cycle related pathways also fits to the observed alterations of miR-132/212 expression in various types of cancer.

Another validated target of miR-132-3p, is RASA1. Downregulation of RASA1 and subsequently neurite outgrowth was observed in various models and is linked to an activation of ERK, RAS and MAPK signaling pathway. Signaling through RAS and MAPK are among the most important mechanisms for cell growth (Hancock et al. 2014; Anand et al. 2010; Antoine-Bertrand et al. 2016; Lei et al. 2015). The involvement of RASA1 also fits to miR-132/212 related observations in cardiovascular diseases and cancer. Interestingly, activation of the ERK1 pathway was also reported to increase miR-132 levels (Chen et al. 2012).

It is remarkable that RAC1, CDC42 and RHOA – three major GTPases controlling cytoskeleton dynamics – are involved in the proposed pathways. The protein ARHGAP32 is a repeatedly validated target of miR-132-3p. Downregulation of ARHGAP32 consequently leads to an upregulation of CDC42, RAC1 and RHOA (Okabe et al. 2003; Moon et al. 2003; Zhao et al. 2003; Nakazawa et al. 2003; Impey et al. 2010). The activation of RAC1 is the most frequently used mechanism to explain the increased neurite length after increased levels of miR-132-3p (Impey et al. 2010; Vo et al. 2005; Wayman et al. 2008). Besides, also the overexpression of CDC42 is described to increase neurite outgrowth (Matsukawa et al. 2018).

On the other hand, the ARHGAP32 target RHOA must be inactivated for a subsequent inactivation of ROCK to increase neurite growth (Matsukawa et al. 2018; Koch et al. 2014). Evidently, the protein interactions depend to a large extent on the model employed. In their model of hippocampal neuron cultures, Impey and colleagues did not observe altered RHOA levels neither after overexpression of miR-132-3p nor after specific downregulation of ARHGAP32.

Moreover, the activation of RHOA by ARHGAP32 downregulation might also be vanished by the simultaneous activation of CDC42, which is a known RHOA inhibitor (Matsukawa et al. 2018). RHOA might further be inactivated via inactivation of ARHGEF11, which is a predicted target both for miR-132-3p and miR-212-3p and was also downregulated for both miRNAs in SWATH-MS. Furthermore, downregulation of ARHGEF11 was shown to improve neurite growth via inactivation of RHOA (Lin et al. 2011).

The proposed pathways and mechanisms induced by miR-132/212 are based on experiments and literature research in very specific and often highly artificial models. Results can dependent on the model, the disease and on the technique of miRNA transfection, transduction or knockout. Nevertheless, the summarized results indicate that the miR-132/212 cluster – and especially miR-132-3p – which was predominantly investigated – regulated some of the most important pathways for cell growth, cell proliferation and cell survival. This fits very well to the upregulation of miR-132-3p in maturing PMN initially observed by Roser and colleagues (Roser 2016; Roser et al. 2018b).

5.7 miR-132-3p and miR-212-3p show different effects in neurite growth and regeneration experiments

Interestingly, miR-132-3p was the only miRNA which induced significant effects in the performed ICC experiments. As the sequence of both miRNAs is very similar and they even share an identical seed sequence – which is especially important for binding to the target mRNA – one would generally assume a large overlap of targets and similar effects. However, miR-212-3p as well as a combination of miR-132-3p and miR-212-3p did not alter neurite growth, regeneration or cell survival after MPP^+ treatment. In the proteomics analysis miR-132-3p regulated more targets and GO clusters than miR-212-3p and significantly affected three KEGG pathways. A series of different hypothesis aims to explain this interesting observation.

First, we hypothesize that the effects on neurite growth of miR-132-3p are intimately linked to a downregulation of ARHGAP32, which is neither a predicted target of miR-212-3p nor was its expression significantly changed in the present experiments. The unchanged levels of ARHGAP32, MECP2 and other miR-132-3p affected pathways discussed earlier, could thus explain why neurite growth is not altered in miR-212-3p treated PMN. However, the neutralization of miR-132-3p effects on growth and regeneration in the co-transfected condition drew our attention to a possible combinatorial regulation in the effects of the two miRNAs.

On the one hand, the findings in the co-transfected condition could be related to the treatment with an increased amount of miRNA mimics. As the cells are transfected with double the amount of miRNA mimics in that condition, possible disturbances of the miRNA machinery might occur. Moreover, even though both miRNAs are transcribed together, the mature miRNA strands can be expressed differently. In studies with hippocampal neuron cultures miR-132-3p was the only mature miRNA strand from the miR-132/212 locus (Magill et al. 2010). Thus, it could be that unexplored mechanisms selecting the miR-132-3p strand as the only active mature miRNA strand, also reduce the effects of transfected miR-212-3p mimics. Measurement by qPCR of miR-212-3p levels 24 hours after transfection showed massively increased levels compared to NC. Although, considering the large amount of transfected miRNA mimics (relatively to endogenous levels) and the miR-212-3p mediated effects in SWATH-MS and Western blot, a specific counter regulation against transfected miR-212-3p is not very likely.

On the other hand, it is also imaginable that miR-212-3p induces pathways to limit effects of miR-132-3p as a sort of miRNA cluster inherent counter regulation. A possible mechanism of miR-212-3p counter regulation could be the repression of EPHA5. In the present SWATH-MS and Western blots EPHA5 was downregulated in PMN transfected with mimics of miR-212-3p. It is also a predicted target of both miRNAs. Signaling via the Ephrin tyrosine kinase receptors is involved in axon guidance by inducing a collapse or repulsion of the growing neurite.

Several studies report improved neurite growth after downregulation of EPHA5 and increased EPHA5 signaling was shown to decrease the average neurite length in cortical neurons (Gao et al. 1998). Moreover, investigations in retinal ganglion cells (RGC) showed that EPHA5 signaling led to increased RHOA activity and decreased RAC1 activity – the opposite regulation of the growth improving effects related to miR-132-3p. Interestingly, inhibition of ROCK prevented the typical EPHA5 induced growth cone collapse in the same experimental setting (Wahl et al. 2000). Other Ephrin receptor isoforms like EPHB2 were also reported to inactivate the RAS-MAPK pathway via an activation of RASA1 (Elowe et al. 2001). According to these reports, decreased EPHA5 receptor expression – like observed for miR-212-3p in Western blot and SWATH-MS – would rather lead to increased neurite outgrowth.

However, in other studies EPHA5 signaling was reported to be beneficial for neurite growth. In a similar model of TH positive sympathetic neuroblast, it could be demonstrated that EPHA5 signaling had a reverse effect and could improve neurite growth (Gao et al. 2000).

Moreover, the need of EPHA5 activation (by its ephrin-A5 ligand) for dopaminergic axon outgrowth was demonstrated in rat PMN (Cooper et al. 2009). According to the observations of the two above mentioned studies., the decreased levels of EPHA5 observed in SWATH-MS and Western blot could lead to decreased neurite growth and could thus be a possible explanation for the neutralized effects of miR-132-3p in the co-transfected condition. Following this hypothesis, however, one could even expect decreased neurite growth and regeneration in the miR-212-3p transfected condition.

Notwithstanding, the present experiments did only measure expression of the EPHA5 receptor and did not investigate whether the observed reduction of the EPHA5 receptor also leads to reduced EPHA5 activity and downstream signaling. Thus, it would be necessary to further examine EPHA5 effects in the present model. Activity of EPHA5 should be measured as well as expression levels of possible downstream targets such as RHOA and RAC1 in EPHA5 siRNA treated cells. Furthermore, evaluation of neurite growth and regeneration would be ideally repeated with EPHA5 siRNA and with miR-132-3p plus EPHA5 siRNA treated conditions. Thereby, one could test whether miR-212-3p induced EPHA5 downregulation is indeed involved in the neutralization of miR-132-3p effects on neurite growth and regeneration.

As discussed above, the present experiments cannot explain the underlying mechanisms of the neutralization of miR-132-3p effects on neurite growth and regeneration in the co-transfected condition. Literature compilation on the topic showed that the majority of studies focused exclusively on miR-132-3p. On the other hand, miR-212-3p is often mentioned in the context of knockout models, where the whole miRNA locus was deleted, but is rarely investigated separately. Consequently, the number of validated targets is much larger for miR-132-3p than for miR-212-3p (Wanet et al. 2012). A small RNA sequencing of miR-132/212 overexpressing mice showed much more regulated mRNA for miR-132 (928) than for miR-212 (58) (Hansen et al. 2016). To a lesser extent, this tendency was also observed in the present SWATH-MS and underlines the dominance of miR-132-3p not only in literature. Taken together, the different effects of the miRNA mimics used here, follow the pattern of other scientific publications. Furthermore, they indicate a strong dominance of the miR-132 strand in the mediation of effects related to the miR-132/212. However, this might be a biased impression, as most studies exclusively investigated the miR-132-3p strand. Several hypotheses were discussed which lead to the observed effects and more experiments need to be performed to determine the underlying mechanisms. Limitations of the miRNA-mimic model as well as a mechanistic counter regulation possibly involving EPHA5 are among the potential causes of the observed effects.

5.8 Concluding remarks

miRNAs are investigated in many different models and diseases. As parts of the epigenetic machinery their transcription and activity can be influenced by the environment and these alterations can even be transmitted to following generations. This discovery has opened new fields for the investigation of etiology, risk factors and pathogenesis of diseases.

Highly interesting is the use of miRNAs as therapeutic agents or targets. A lot of studies with animal models suggested possible beneficial effects of miRNA replacement or inhibition. For instance, replacement of AAV transduced miR-132 improved the survival in a mice model of HD (Fukuoka et al. 2018). Furthermore, replacement of miR-7 is discussed as (possibly disease modifying) therapy for PD patients. The miRNA targets α-synuclein and was also shown to have neuroprotective effects which could not be confirmed in the experiments of this study (Titze-de-Almeida and Titze-de-Almeida 2018).

Exogenous replacement of miRNA or their targeted downregulation e.g. via siRNA would be especially practical if the miRNA alteration would be the actual origin of the disease. Even though manipulation of miRNA levels can have beneficial effects in several models as discussed earlier, they always target incalculable many mRNA. Referring to the mechanisms regulated by miR-132-3p with enhanced cell survival or cell growth, introducing exogenous miRNA mimics would probably also mean to elevate the risk of cancer genesis. This would mean an intolerable side effect, especially in relatively slow progressing ND like PD. Moreover, miR-132-3p targets NURR1 – a protein which is found downregulated in PD patients and is discussed as a putative replacement agent in PD therapy. Thus, it is unclear whether an overexpression (improving growth and regeneration) or downregulation of miR-132-3p (rescuing NURR1) would be more promising for PD patients (Decressac et al. 2013).

Nevertheless, a review from 2017 listed four inhibitors and three mimics of miRNA which made it to clinical phase I or even phase II trials. Treatment indications are different neoplasia, scleroderma and Hepatitis C (Rupaimoole and Slack 2017). More applications for patents try to protect the idea of "miRNA as novel therapeutic targets and diagnostic biomarkers" in PD (in particular the miR-132/212 cluster, WO2014018650) and specifically for the miR-132/212 cluster in cardiac disorders (WO2013034653A1). Although, an evaluation of the first named patent soberly underlined the unsolved problems and obstacles, patents and possibly following financial support can help to continue the promising research on miRNA in neurodegenerative diseases (Hesse and Arenz 2014). In this context, the miR-132/212 was demonstrated to have a broad influence on various important cell signaling pathways.

6 Summary

All experiments were performed with the idea of gaining more knowledge on the effects of the miR-132/212 cluster in dopaminergic PMN. Therefore, PMN were transfected with the two mature strands miR-132-3p and miR-212-3p and their influence on growth, regeneration and neuroprotection was analyzed. Furthermore, the underlying mechanisms of the effects of these miRNAs were investigated to better understand how neurite growth and regeneration processes are regulated and to possibly identify interesting proteins controlling this mechanism for future therapeutic use. Based on these results, miR-132-3p and miR-212-3p were to evaluate as putative therapeutic agents or targets in PD.

The experiments showed that only increased levels of miR-132-3p improved neurite growth and neurite regeneration in dopaminergic PMN. However, transfection with miR-212-3p or with both miRNAs combined did not alter growth respectively regeneration compared to NC siRNA treatment. None of the three experimental conditions could protect dopaminergic neurons from MPP^+ toxicity. SWATH-MS indicated an involvement of major growth regulating pathways. Several growth, maturation or regeneration related proteins were demonstrated to be regulated by the applied miRNA transfection in Western blot analysis of PMN lysates. An extensive literature research indicated more targets of the two miRNAs and possibly related pathways investigated in other models but related to the observations in PMN.

On the one hand, improved growth or regeneration as induced by increased levels of miR-132-3p are possibly beneficial in diseases like PD. On the other hand, other targets of this miRNA were reported to be essential and probably even lacking in PD patients' dopaminergic neurons and must thus not be downregulated by overexpression of the miRNA. Taken together, a generally beneficial effect of increased levels of these miRNAs in PD or other diseases is doubtful. However, identification of targets and pathways under their control can extend the knowledge on neuron maturation and regeneration possibly leading to interesting targets for new therapeutic approaches.

7 Appendix

Table A1 The 15 most significantly affected KEGG pathways in mice according to seed-sequence-based target prediction of miR-132/212 targets by targetscan.org

KEGG pathway Term		p-Value
mmu05200	Pathways in cancer	7.1E-6
mmu05215	Prostate cancer	1.0E-4
mmu05213	Endometrial cancer	2.1E-4
mmu04550	Signaling pathways regulating pluripotency of stem cells	4.6E-4
mmu04350	TGF-beta signaling pathway	5.0E-4
mmu05210	Colorectal cancer	6.4E-4
mmu04360	Axon guidance	1.3E-3
mmu05217	Basal cell carcinoma	1.9E-3
mmu04390	Hippo signaling pathway	3.6E-3
mmu04520	Adherens junction	6.8E-3
mmu04068	FoxO signaling pathway	6.9E-3
mmu04010	MAPL signaling pathway	8.9E-3
mmu04310	Wnt signaling pathway	9.0E-3
mmu05221	Acute myeloid leukemia	1.4E-2
mmu04012	ErbB signaling pathway	1.5E-2

Table A2 Overlap of regulated targets from SWATH-MS and targets predicted by three different target prediction databases

Predicted and regulated targets of miR-132-3p			Predicted and regulated targets of miR-212-3p		
targetscan.org (5)	**microrna.org (16)**	**mirwalk.org (67)**	**targetscan.org (3)**	**microrna.org (17)**	**mirwalk.org (65)**
ARHGEF11	ARHGEF11	ADPRH	ARHGEF11	ARHGEF11	AAAS
MAPT	CHCHD3	AP3D1	PAPOLA	CHCHD3	ACTR1B
MECP2	CNTN1	APRT	SRSF1	CLTC	ALB
PAPOLA	CYFIP1	ARHGEF11		DYNC1LI1	ARHGEF11
RRAS2	FYTTD1	ARHGEF40		EPHA5	AU040320
	GNAI1	BAX		GNAI1	CCDC51
	GPM6A	CASP3		HNRNPK	CDC37
	IPO9	CCDC51		NSUN2	CHCHD3
	MAPT	CHCHD3		PAPOLA	CISD2
	NSUN2	CNTN1		PHF3	CLTC
	PAPOLA	CPSF3		PRIM2	D10JHU81E
	PHF3	CSNK2B		RAE1	D630045J12RIK
	PTS	CYFIP1		RBM27	DCTN2
	RRAS2	D10JHU81E		SCAMP1	DDX27
	SRPK2	D630045J12RIK		SRPK2	DDX56
	WDR11	DCTN2		SUB1	DYNC1LI1
		DLG4		TRAFD1	ECHDC1
		ECHDC1			EIF2B4
		ESD			EPHA5
		EXOSC7			EXOSC7
		FYTTD1			FABP3
		GET4			FAM69B

Predicted and regulated targets of miR-132-3p			**Predicted and regulated targets of miR-212-3p**		
targetscan.org (5)	**microrna.org (16)**	**mirwalk.org (67)**	**targetscan.org (3)**	**microrna.org (17)**	**mirwalk.org (65)**
		GNAI1			GLO1
		GPM6A			GNAI1
		GPX4			GPS1
		HSD17B10			HMGB2
		INTS1			HNRNPK
		MAPT			INPP4A
		MDH1			ISOC1
		ME1			MAP1LC3B
		MECP2			MAP4
		MRPL10			ME1
		MSH6			MRPL11
		MYDGF			NDRG3
		NSUN2			NSUN2
		NUMBL			PAF1
		PAPOLA			PAPOLA
		PGM2			PHF3
		PHF3			POR
		PI4K2A			PPP3CA
		POR			PRIM2
		PPP3CA			PSMD8
		PREB			RAE1
		PSMD8			RBM27
		PTS			RPL13
		RAB9			RPL35A
		RAD21			RTCB
		RBMX			SCAMP1
		ROCK2			SCFD2
		RPL35A			SH3GL2
		RRAS2			SLC25A51
		SF3B2			SPTBN2
		SH3GL2			SRPK2
		SLC25A51			SUB1
		SPTBN2			TAX1BP3
		SRPK2			TOM1L2
		STK11			TRAFD1
		STRIP1			TST
		TJP1			UBE2E3
		TOM1L2			WDR61
		TXLNA			YARS
		USP47			YEATS4
		WDR11			YES1
		YARS			ZFP638
		YES1			ZMIZ1
		ZFP638			
		ZMIZ1			

Table A3 Significantly involved GO clusters of targets regulated differentially in SWATH-MS

#	GO-clusters miR-132	p-value	#	GO clusters miR-212	p-value
1	GO:0006886~intracellular protein transport	7.58E-03	1	GO:1904322~cellular response to forskolin	1.03E-03
2	GO:0021692~cerebellar Purkinje cell layer morphogenesis	1.57E-02	2	GO:0006412~translation	5.59E-03
3	GO:0006974~cellular response to DNA damage stimulus	2.33E-02	3	GO:0010501~RNA secondary structure unwinding	1.42E-02
4	GO:0007416~synapse assembly	2.34E-02	4	GO:0006364~rRNA processing	1.44E-02
5	GO:0007266~Rho protein signal transduction	2.43E-02	5	GO:0007067~mitotic nuclear division	2.57E-02
6	GO:0055114~oxidation-reduction process	2.58E-02	6	GO:0006397~mRNA processing	4.12E-02
7	GO:0016192~vesicle-mediated transport	2.60E-02	7	GO:0008033~tRNA processing	4.63E-02
8	GO:0006915~apoptotic process	3.05E-01			
9	GO:0007007~inner mitochondrial membrane organization	3.11E-02			
10	GO:0006108~malate metabolic process	4.13E-02			
11	GO:0010033~response to organic substance	4.59E-02			
12	GO:0043154~negative regulation of cysteine-type endopeptidase activity involved in apoptotic process	4.84E-02			
13	GO:0007399~nervous system development	4.86E-02			

Table A4 Summary of results from SWATH-MS and Western blots and references for the discussed proteins and pathways

Legend: ↓ downregulation; ↑ upregulation ~ unchanged expression + predicted target - not a predicted target

Target (Alias names)	miR-132-3p			miR-212-3p			Results from this book		Reported results	Reference
	Targetscan	microrna	mirwalk	Targetscan	microrna	mirwalk	SWATH-MS	Western blot		
ARHGAP32 (p250GAP, RHG32)	+	+	+	+	+	+	miR-132-3p: ↓ miR-212-3p: ~	miR-132-3p: ↓ miR-212-3p: ~	Target of miR-132-3p	(Vo et al. 2005; Impey et al. 2010; Wayman et al. 2008)
									Inactivates CDC42, RAC1 and RHOA	(Okabe et al. 2003; Moon et al. 2003; Zhao et al. 2003; Nakazawa et al. 2003; Impey et al. 2010)
ARHGEF11 (PDZ-RHOGEF)	+	+	+	+	+	+	miR-132-3p: ↓ miR-212-3p: ↓	---	Inhibition increases neurite outgrowth	(Lin et al. 2011)
									Overexpression decreases spine density	(Mizuki et al. 2016)
									Activates RhoA and subsequently ROCK	(Sai et al. 2014; Wang et al. 2018b)
CDC42	-	-	-	-	-	-	miR-132-3p: ~ miR-212-3p: ~	---	Inactivated by ARHGAP32	(Zhao et al. 2003; Okabe et al. 2003; Nakazawa et al. 2003)
									Inactivates RHOA	(Matsukawa et al. 2018)
EPHA5	-	+	+	-	+	+	miR-132-3p: ~ miR-212-3p: ↓	miR-132-3p: ~ miR-212-3p: ↓	EPHA5 signaling decreases neurite length	(Gao et al. 1998)
									EPHA5 signaling increases neurite length in TH+/dopaminergic neurons	(Gao et al. 2000; Cooper et al. 2009)
									Activates RHOA and inactivates RAC1	(Wahl et al. 2000)

Target (Alias names)	miR-132-3p			miR-212-3p			Results from this book		Reported results	Reference
	Targetscan	microrna	mirwalk	Targetscan	microrna	mirwalk	SWATH-MS	Western blot		
FOXO3	+	+	-	+	+	+	not detected	---	Target of miR-132, Target of the miR-132/212 cluster	(Mehta et al. 2015; Wong et al. 2013)
									Inhibited by the PI3K downstream target AKT	(Santo et al. 2013)
									Downregulation of FOXO3 has anti-apoptotic / pro survival effects and improves neurite growth and regeneration	(Roser et al. 2018b; Wong et al. 2013; Wang et al. 2013a)
MECP2	+	-	+	+	-	-	miR-132-3p: ↓ miR-212-3p: ~	miR-132-3p: ↓ miR-212-3p: ~	Target of miR-132-3p and miR-212-3p	(Im et al. 2010; Wada et al. 2010; Klein et al. 2007)
PTEN	+	+	+	+	+	-	not detected	---	Target of miR-132-3p, Inhibition works anti-apoptotic	(Jin et al. 2012; Gu et al. 2018; Wong et al. 2013)
									Activated by ROCK	(Li et al. 2005)
									Inhibition leads to increased neurite growth and specially to enhanced neurite regeneration	(Park et al. 2008; Ohtake et al. 2015)
RAC1	-	-	-	-	-	-	not detected	---	Inactivated by ARHGAP32	(Zhao et al. 2003; Okabe et al. 2003; Moon et al. 2003; Impey et al. 2010)
									Overexpression increases neurite outgrowth	(Matsukawa et al. 2018)

Target (Alias names)	miR-132-3p			miR-212-3p			Results from this book		Reported results	Reference
	Targetscan	microrna	mirwalk	Targetscan	microrna	mirwalk	SWATH-MS	Western blot		
RASA1 (p120GAP)	+	-	+	+	-	-	miR-132-3p: ~ miR-212-3p: ~	---	Target of miR-132-3p	(Hancock et al. 2014; Anand et al. 2010; Antoine-Bertrand et al. 2016; Lei et al. 2015)
RHOA	-	-	-	-	-	+	miR-132-3p: ~ miR-212-3p: ~	---	Activated by ARHGEF11	(Wang et al. 2018b)
									Inactivated by ARHGAP32	(Okabe et al. 2003; Moon et al. 2003; Nakazawa et al. 2003)
									Inactivated by CDC42	(Matsukawa et al. 2018)
									Downregulation of RHOA leads to neurite outgrowth	(Luo 2000; Govek et al. 2005; Hall and Lalli 2010)
									Activator of ROCK, inhibits neurite outgrowth	(Nakayama et al. 2000)
ROCK2	-	-	+	-	-	+	miR-132-3p: ↓ miR-212-3p: ~	miR-132-3p: ~ miR-212-3p: ~	ROCK inhibition leads to increased neurite growth	(Nakayama et al. 2000; Koch et al. 2014)
MAPT (TAU)	+	+	+	+	+	+	miR-132-3p: ↑ miR-212-3p: ~	---	Tau is a target of miR-132-3p and miR-132/212 deficiency promotes tau aggregation	(Smith et al. 2015)
									Overexpression increases neurite growth	(Zuo et al. 2016)
									Tau deficiency decreased neurite growth	(Dawson et al. 2001)
TAX1BP3	-	-	-	-	+	+	miR-132-3p: ↑ miR-212-3p: ↑	miR-132-3p: ~ miR-212-3p: ~	Inactivates RHOA via rhotekin	(Matsukawa et al. 2018)---

8 References

Agarwal V, Bell GW, Nam J-W, Bartel DP (2015): Predicting effective microRNA target sites in mammalian mRNAs. Elife 4, e05005

Alexander RP, Fang G, Rozowsky J, Snyder M, Gerstein MB (2010): Annotating non-coding regions of the genome. Nat Rev Genet 11, 559–571

Alvarez-Saavedra M, Antoun G, Yanagiya A, Oliva-Hernandez R, Cornejo-Palma D, Perez-Iratxeta C, Sonenberg N, Cheng HYM (2011): miRNA-132 orchestrates chromatin remodeling and translational control of the circadian clock. Hum Mol Genet 20, 731–751

Ameres SL, Zamore PD (2013): Diversifying microRNA sequence and function. Nat Rev Mol Cell Biol 14, 475–488

Anand S, Majeti BK, Acevedo LM, Murphy EA, Mukthavaram R, Scheppke L, Huang M, Shields DJ, Lindquist JN, Lapinski PE et al. (2010): MicroRNA-132-mediated loss of p120RasGAP activates the endothelium to facilitate pathological angiogenesis. Nat Med 16, 909–914

Angot E, Steiner JA, Hansen C, Li JY, Brundin P (2010): Are synucleinopathies prion-like disorders? Lancet Neurol 9, 1128–1138

Antoine-Bertrand J, Duquette PM, Alchini R, Kennedy TE, Fournier AE, Lamarche-Vane N (2016): p120RasGAP Protein Mediates Netrin-1 Protein-induced Cortical Axon Outgrowth and Guidance. J Biol Chem 291, 4589–4602

Atanassov I, Urlaub H (2013): Increased proteome coverage by combining PAGE and peptide isoelectric focusing: Comparative study of gel-based separation approaches. Proteomics 13, 2947–2955

Aten S, Hansen KF, Hoyt KR, Obrietan K (2016): The miR-132/212 locus: A complex regulator of neuronal plasticity, gene expression and cognition. RNA Dis 3, e1375

Aten S, Page CE, Kalidindi A, Wheaton K, Niraula A, Godbout JP, Hoyt K, Obrietan K (2018): miR-132/212 is induced by stress and its dysregulation triggers anxiety-related behavior. Neuropharmacology 21, 2323–2329

Beal MF, Oakes D, Shoulson I, Henchcliffe C, Galpern WR, Haas R, Juncos JL, Nutt JG, Voss TS, Ravina B et al. (2014): A randomized clinical trial of high-dosage coenzyme Q10 in early Parkinson disease: No evidence of benefit. JAMA Neurol 71, 543–552

Benito E, Kerimoglu C, Ramachandran B, Pena-Centeno T, Jain G, Stilling RM, Islam MR, Capece V, Zhou Q, Edbauer D et al. (2018): RNA-Dependent Intergenerational Inheritance of Enhanced Synaptic Plasticity after Environmental Enrichment. Cell Rep 23, 546–554

Bentley P, Sharma P: Neurological disorders – epilepsy, Parkinson's disease and multiple sclerosis. In: Bennett PN, Brown MJ, Sharma P (Eds.): Clinical pharmacology. 11th edition; Elsevier, Edinburgh 2012, 349–370

Bernheimer H, Birkmayer W, Hornykiewicz O, Jellinger K, Seitelberger F (1973): Brain dopamine and the syndromes of Parkinson and Huntington - Clinical, morphological and neurochemical correlations. J. Neurol. Sci. 20, 415–455

Bertler A, Rosengren E (1959): Occurrence and distribution of dopamine in brain and other tissues. Experientia 15, 10–11

Bertler A, Rosengren E (1966): Possible role of brain dopamine. Pharmacol Rev 18, 769–773

Betel D, Wilson M, Gabow A, Marks DS, Sander C (2008): The microRNA.org resource: Targets and expression. Nucleic Acids Res 36, D149-D153

Betel D, Koppal A, Agius P, Sander C, Leslie C (2010): Comprehensive modeling of microRNA targets predicts functional non-conserved and non-canonical sites. Genome Biol. 11, R90

Bhattacherjee A, Mu Y, Winter MK, Knapp JR, Eggimann LS, Gunewardena SS, Kobayashi K, Kato S, Krizsan-Agbas D, Smith PG (2017): Neuronal cytoskeletal gene dysregulation and mechanical hypersensitivity in a rat model of Rett syndrome. Proc Natl Acad Sci U S A 114, E6952-E6961

Bird A (2007): Perceptions of epigenetics. Nature 447, 396–398

Blizzard CA, Haas MA, Vickers JC, Dickson TC (2007): Cellular dynamics underlying regeneration of damaged axons differs from initial axon development. Eur J Neurosci 26, 1100–1108

Braak H, Del Tredici K, Rub U, de Vos, Rob A. I., Jansen Steur ENH, Braak E (2003): Staging of brain pathology related to sporadic Parkinson's disease. Neurobiol Aging 24, 197–211

Brennicke A, Marchfelder A, Binder S (1999): RNA editing. FEMS Microbiol Rev 23, 297–316

Burbulla LF, Song P, Mazzulli JR, Zampese E, Wong YC, Jeon S, Santos DP, Blanz J, Obermaier CD, Strojny C et al. (2017): Dopamine oxidation mediates mitochondrial and lysosomal dysfunction in Parkinson's disease. Science 357, 1255–1261

Burgos K, Malenica I, Metpally R, Courtright A, Rakela B, Beach T, Shill H, Adler C, Sabbagh M, Villa S et al. (2014): Profiles of extracellular miRNA in cerebrospinal fluid and serum from patients with Alzheimer's and Parkinson's diseases correlate with disease status and features of pathology. PLoS One 9, e94839

Burke RE, O'Malley K (2013): Axon degeneration in Parkinson's disease. Exp Neurol 246, 72–83

Byeon H-E, Jeon JY, Kim HJ, Kim DJ, Lee K-W, Kang Y, Han SJ (2017): MicroRNA-132 Negatively Regulates Palmitate-Induced NLRP3 Inflammasome Activation through FOXO3 Down-Regulation in THP-1 Cells. Nutrients 9, 1370

Caldi Gomes LA: The effect of increased levels of miR-132 on dopaminergic primary midbrain neurons. Master's book. Göttingen 2016

Carboni E, Tatenhorst L, Tönges L, Barski E, Dambeck V, Bähr M, Lingor P (2017): Deferiprone Rescues Behavioral Deficits Induced by Mild Iron Exposure in a Mouse Model of Alpha-Synuclein Aggregation. Neuromolecular Med 19, 309–321

Chakraborty C, Sharma AR, Sharma G, Doss CGP, Lee S-S (2017): Therapeutic miRNA and siRNA: Moving from Bench to Clinic as Next Generation Medicine. Mol Ther Nucleic Acids 8, 132–143

Chen C, Wirth A, Ponimaskin E (2012): Cdc42: an important regulator of neuronal morphology. Int J Biochem Cell Biol 44, 447–451

Choi DC, Chae Y-J, Kabaria S, Chaudhuri AD, Jain MR, Li H, Mouradian MM, Junn E (2014): MicroRNA-7 protects against 1-methyl-4-phenylpyridinium-induced cell death by targeting RelA. J Neurosci 34, 12725–12737

Chu Y, Kordower JH (2010): Lewy body pathology in fetal grafts. Ann N Y Acad Sci 1184, 55–67

Clarke CE (2007): Parkinson's disease. BMJ 335, 441–445

Cooper MA, Kobayashi K, Zhou R (2009): Ephrin-A5 regulates the formation of the ascending midbrain dopaminergic pathways. Dev Neurobiol 69, 36–46

Coppede F (2012): Genetics and epigenetics of Parkinson's disease. Scientific World Journal 2012, 489830

Corsini GU, Zuddas A, Bonuccelli U, Schinelli S, Kopin IJ (1987): 1-Methyl-4-phenyl-1,2,3,6-tetrahydropyridine (MPTP) neurotoxicity in mice is enhanced by ethanol or acetaldehyde. Life Sci 40, 827–832

Cox J, Mann M (2008): MaxQuant enables high peptide identification rates, individualized p.p.b.-range mass accuracies and proteome-wide protein quantification. Nat Biotechnol 26, 1367–1372

Dauer W, Przedborski S (2003): Parkinson's disease: mechanisms and models. Neuron 39, 889–909

Davis GC, Williams AC, Markey SP, Ebert MH, Caine ED, Reichert CM, Kopin IJ (1979): Chronic parkinsonism secondary to intravenous injection of meperidine analogues. Psychiatry Research 1, 249–254

Dawson HN, Ferreira A, Eyster MV, Ghoshal N, Binder LI, Vitek MP (2001): Inhibition of neuronal maturation in primary hippocampal neurons from tau deficient mice. J Cell Sci 114, 1179–1187

de Lau LML, Breteler MMB (2006): Epidemiology of Parkinson's disease. Lancet Neurol 5, 525–535

de Rijk MC, Breteler MM, Graveland GA, Ott A, Grobbee DE, van der Meche FG, Hofman A (1995): Prevalence of Parkinson's disease in the elderly: the Rotterdam Study. Neurology 45, 2143–2146 de Rijk MC, Launer LJ, Berger K, Breteler MM, Dartigues JF, Baldereschi M, Fratiglioni L, Lobo A, Martinez-Lage J, Trenkwalder C et al. (2000): Prevalence of Parkinson's disease in Europe: A collaborative study of population-based cohorts. Neurologic Diseases in the Elderly Research Group. Neurology 54, 21-23

Decressac M, Kadkhodaei B, Mattsson B, Laguna A, Perlmann T, Björklund A (2012): α-Synuclein-induced down-regulation of Nurr1 disrupts GDNF signaling in nigral dopamine neurons. Sci Transl Med 4, 163ra156

Decressac M, Volakakis N, Björklund A, Perlmann T (2013): NURR1 in Parkinson disease--from pathogenesis to therapeutic potential. Nat Rev Neurol 9, 629–636

Deeb W, Hu W, Almeida L, Patterson A, Martinez-Ramirez D, Wagle Shukla A (2016): Benign tremulous Parkinsonism: A unique entity or another facet of Parkinson's disease? Transl Neurodegener 5, 10

Dexter DT, Jenner P (2013): Parkinson disease: From pathology to molecular disease mechanisms. Free Radic Biol Med 62, 132–144

Dias BG, Ressler KJ (2013): Parental olfactory experience influences behavior and neural structure in subsequent generations. Nat Neurosci 17, 89-96

Dickson DW, Braak H, Duda JE, Duyckaerts C, Gasser T, Halliday GM, Hardy J, Leverenz JB, Del Tredici K, Wszolek ZK et al. (2009): Neuropathological assessment of Parkinson's disease: Refining the diagnostic criteria. Lancet Neurology 8, 1150–1157

Didiano D, Hobert O (2006): Perfect seed pairing is not a generally reliable predictor for miRNA-target interactions. Nat Struct Mol Biol 13, 849–851

Dölle C, Flønes I, Nido GS, Miletic H, Osuagwu N, Kristoffersen S, Lilleng PK, Larsen JP, Tysnes O-B, Haugarvoll K et al. (2016): Defective mitochondrial DNA homeostasis in the substantia nigra in Parkinson disease. Nat Commun 7, 13548

Donadio V, Incensi A, Leta V, Giannoccaro MP, Scaglione C, Martinelli P, Capellari S, Avoni P, Baruzzi A, Liguori R (2014): Skin nerve α-synuclein deposits: A biomarker for idiopathic Parkinson disease. Neurology 82, 1362–1369

Doppler K, Jentschke H-M, Schulmeyer L, Vadasz D, Janzen A, Luster M, Höffken H, Mayer G, Brumberg J, Booij J et al. (2017): Dermal phospho-alpha-synuclein deposits confirm REM sleep behaviour disorder as prodromal Parkinson's disease. Acta Neuropathol 133, 535–545

Dweep H, Gretz N (2015): miRWalk2.0: A comprehensive atlas of microRNA-target interactions. Nat Methods 12, 697

Eggers C, Pedrosa DJ, Kahraman D, Maier F, Lewis CJ, Fink GR, Schmidt M, Timmermann L (2012): Parkinson subtypes progress differently in clinical course and imaging pattern. PLoS One 7, e46813

Elowe S, Holland SJ, Kulkarni S, Pawson T (2001): Downregulation of the Ras-mitogen-activated protein kinase pathway by the EphB2 receptor tyrosine kinase is required for ephrin-induced neurite retraction. Mol Cell Biol 21, 7429–7441

ENCODE Project Consortium (2012): An integrated encyclopedia of DNA elements in the human genome. Nature 489, 57–74

Fahn S (2005): Does levodopa slow or hasten the rate of progression of Parkinson's disease? J Neurol 252 Suppl 4, IV37-IV42

Feng J, Nestler EJ (2010): MeCP2 and drug addiction. Nat Neurosci 13, 1039–1041

Fereshtehnejad S-M, Romenets SR, Anang JBM, Latreille V, Gagnon J-F, Postuma RB (2015): New Clinical Subtypes of Parkinson Disease and Their Longitudinal Progression: A Prospective Cohort Comparison With Other Phenotypes. JAMA Neurol 72, 863–873

Finkelstein DI, Hare DJ, Billings JL, Sedjahtera A, Nurjono M, Arthofer E, George S, Culvenor JG, Bush AI, Adlard PA (2016): Clioquinol Improves Cognitive, Motor Function, and Microanatomy of the Alpha-Synuclein hA53T Transgenic Mice. ACS Chem Neurosci 7, 119–129

Fire A, Xu S, Montgomery MK, Kostas SA, Driver SE, Mello CC (1998): Potent and specific genetic interference by double-stranded RNA in Caenorhabditis elegans. Nature 391, 806–811

Fischer A (2014): Epigenetic memory: the Lamarckian brain. EMBO J 33, 945–967

Fischer A (2016): Environmental enrichment as a method to improve cognitive function. What can we learn from animal models? Neuroimage 131, 42–47

Flønes IH, Fernandez-Vizarra E, Lykouri M, Brakedal B, Skeie GO, Miletic H, Lilleng PK, Alves G, Tysnes O-B, Haugarvoll K et al. (2018): Neuronal complex I deficiency occurs throughout the Parkinson's disease brain, but is not associated with neurodegeneration or mitochondrial DNA damage. Acta Neuropathol 135, 409–425

Freed CR, Greene PE, Breeze RE, Tsai WY, DuMouchel W, Kao R, Dillon S, Winfield H, Culver S, Trojanowski JQ et al. (2001): Transplantation of embryonic dopamine neurons for severe Parkinson's disease. N Engl J Med 344, 710–719

Fuentes EO, Leemhuis J, Stark GB, Lang EM (2008): Rho kinase inhibitors Y27632 and H1152 augment neurite extension in the presence of cultured Schwann cells. J Brachial Plex Peripher Nerve Inj 3, 19

Fukuoka M, Takahashi M, Fujita H, Chiyo T, Popiel HA, Watanabe S, Furuya H, Murata M, Wada K, Okada T et al. (2018): Supplemental Treatment for Huntington's Disease with miR-132 that Is Deficient in Huntington's Disease Brain. Mol Ther Nucleic Acids 11, 79–90

Gage H, Storey L (2004): Rehabilitation for Parkinson's disease: A systematic review of available evidence. Clin Rehabil 18, 463–482

Gao PP, Yue Y, Zhang JH, Cerretti DP, Levitt P, Zhou R (1998): Regulation of thalamic neurite outgrowth by the Eph ligand ephrin-A5: Implications in the development of thalamocortical projections. Proc Natl Acad Sci U S A 95, 5329–5334

Gao P-P, Sun C-H, Zhou X-F, DiCicco-Bloom E, Zhou R (2000): Ephrins stimulate or inhibit neurite outgrowth and survival as a function of neuronal cell type. Journal of Neuroscience Research 60, 427–436

Gasser T, Hardy J, Mizuno Y (2011): Milestones in PD genetics. Mov Disord 26, 1042–1048

Gerlach M, Riederer P, Przuntek H, Youdim MBH (1991): MPTP mechanisms of neurotoxicity and their implications for Parkinson's disease. European Journal of Pharmacology: Molecular Pharmacology 208, 273–286

Giasson BI, Lee VM-Y (2003): Are ubiquitination pathways central to Parkinson's disease? Cell 114, 1–8

Gibney ER, Nolan CM (2010): Epigenetics and gene expression. Heredity (Edinb) 105, 4–13

Goedert M, Spillantini MG, Del Tredici K, Braak H (2013): 100 years of Lewy pathology. Nat Rev Neurol 9, 13–24

Goetz CG (2011): The history of Parkinson's disease: early clinical descriptions and neurological therapies. Cold Spring Harb Perspect Med 1, a008862

Govek E-E, Newey SE, van Aelst L (2005): The role of the Rho GTPases in neuronal development. Genes Dev 19, 1–49

Grimes DA, Han F, Panisset M, Racacho L, Xiao F, Zou R, Westaff K, Bulman DE (2006): Translated mutation in the Nurr1 gene as a cause for Parkinson's disease. Mov Disord 21, 906–909

Gui Y, Liu H, Zhang L, Lv W, Hu X (2015): Altered microRNA profiles in cerebrospinal fluid exosome in Parkinson disease and Alzheimer disease. Oncotarget 6, 37043–37053

Gu Y, Cai R, Zhang C, Xue Y, Pan Y, Wang J, Zhang Z (2018): miR-132-3p boosts caveolae-mediated transcellular transport in glioma endothelial cells by targeting PTEN/PI3K/PKB/Src/Cav-1 signaling pathway. FASEB J, 441-454

Hadar A, Milanesi E, Walczak M, Puzianowska-Kuźnicka M, Kuźnicki J, Squassina A, Niola P, Chillotti C, Attems J, Gozes I et al. (2018): SIRT1, miR-132 and miR-212 link human longevity to Alzheimer's Disease. Sci Rep 8, 8465

Hall A, Lalli G (2010): Rho and Ras GTPases in axon growth, guidance, and branching. Cold Spring Harb Perspect Biol 2, a001818

Halliday GM, Holton JL, Revesz T, Dickson DW (2011): Neuropathology underlying clinical variability in patients with synucleinopathies. Acta Neuropathol 122, 187–204

Hancock ML, Preitner N, Quan J, Flanagan JG (2014): MicroRNA-132 Is Enriched in Developing Axons, Locally Regulates Rasa1 mRNA, and Promotes Axon Extension. J Neurosci 34, 66–78

Hanna J, Hossain GS, Kocerha J (2019): The Potential for microRNA Therapeutics and Clinical Research. Front Genet 10, 478

Hansen KF, Sakamoto K, Wayman GA, Impey S, Obrietan K (2010): Transgenic miR132 alters neuronal spine density and impairs novel object recognition memory. PLoS One 5, e15497

Hansen KF, Karelina K, Sakamoto K, Wayman GA, Impey S, Obrietan K (2013): miRNA-132: a dynamic regulator of cognitive capacity. Brain Struct Funct 218, 817–831

Hansen KF, Sakamoto K, Aten S, Snider KH, Loeser J, Hesse AM, Page CE, Pelz C, Arthur JSC, Impey S et al. (2016): Targeted deletion of miR-132/-212 impairs memory and alters the hippocampal transcriptome. Learn Mem 23, 61–71

Hasbani DM, Perez FA, Palmiter RD, O'Malley KL (2005): Dopamine depletion does not protect against acute 1-methyl-4-phenyl-1,2,3,6-tetrahydropyridine toxicity in vivo. J Neurosci 25, 9428–9433

Hastings TG (2009): The role of dopamine oxidation in mitochondrial dysfunction: implications for Parkinson's disease. J Bioenerg Biomembr 41, 469–472

Hawkes CH, Del Tredici K, Braak H (2007): Parkinson's disease: A dual-hit hypothesis. Neuropathol Appl Neurobiol 33, 599–614

Heard E, Martienssen RA (2014): Transgenerational epigenetic inheritance: myths and mechanisms. Cell 157, 95–109

Heman-Ackah SM, Hallegger M, Rao MS, Wood MJA (2013): RISC in PD: the impact of microRNAs in Parkinson's disease cellular and molecular pathogenesis. Front Mol Neurosci 6, 40

Hernandez-Rapp J, Smith PY, Filali M, Goupil C, Planel E, Magill ST, Goodman RH, Hebert SS (2015): Memory formation and retention are affected in adult miR-132/212 knockout mice. Behav Brain Res 287, 15–26

Herrington TM, Cheng JJ, Eskandar EN (2016): Mechanisms of deep brain stimulation. J Neurophysiol 115, 19–38

Hesse M, Arenz C (2014): miRNAs as novel therapeutic targets and diagnostic biomarkers for Parkinson's disease: A patent evaluation of WO2014018650. Expert Opin Ther Pat 24, 1271–1276

Houwing S, Kamminga LM, Berezikov E, Cronembold D, Girard A, van den Elst H, Filippov DV, Blaser H, Raz E, Moens CB et al. (2007): A role for Piwi and piRNAs in germ cell maintenance and transposon silencing in Zebrafish. Cell 129, 69–82

Huang DW, Sherman BT, Tan Q, Kir J, Liu D, Bryant D, Guo Y, Stephens R, Baseler MW, Lane HC et al. (2007): DAVID Bioinformatics Resources: Expanded annotation database and novel algorithms to better extract biology from large gene lists. Nucleic Acids Res 35, W169-175

Huang DW, Sherman BT, Lempicki RA (2009): Systematic and integrative analysis of large gene lists using DAVID bioinformatics resources. Nat Protoc 4, 44–57

Im H-I, Hollander JA, Bali P, Kenny PJ (2010): MeCP2 controls BDNF expression and cocaine intake through homeostatic interactions with microRNA-212. Nat Neurosci 13, 1120–1127

Impey S, Davare M, Lesiak A, Fortin D, Ando H, Varlamova O, Obrietan K, Soderling TR, Goodman RH, Wayman GA (2010): An activity-induced microRNA controls dendritic spine formation by regulating Rac1-PAK signaling. Mol Cell Neurosci 43, 146–156

Iwaki H, Ando R, Miyaue N, Tada S, Tsujii T, Yabe H, Nishikawa N, Nagai M, Nomoto M (2017): One year safety and efficacy of inosine to increase the serum urate level for patients with Parkinson's disease in Japan. Journal of the Neurological Sciences 383, 75–78

Janetzky B, Hauck S, Youdim MB, Riederer P, Jellinger K, Pantucek F, Zöchling R, Boissl KW, Reichmann H (1994): Unaltered aconitase activity, but decreased complex I activity in substantia nigra pars compacta of patients with Parkinson's disease. Neuroscience Letters 169, 126–128

Jankovic J: Parkinson Disease and Other Movement Disorders. In: Daroff RB, Jankovic J, Mazziotta JC, Pomeroy SL (Eds.): Bradley's Neurology in Clinical Practice. 7th edition; Elsevier, London 2015, 1422–1440

Jin W, Reddy MA, Chen Z, Putta S, Lanting L, Kato M, Park JT, Chandra M, Wang C, Tangirala RK et al. (2012): Small RNA Sequencing Reveals MicroRNAs That Modulate Angiotensin II Effects in Vascular Smooth Muscle Cells*. J Biol Chem 287, 15672–15683

Josephs KA, Matsumoto JY, Ahlskog JE (2006): Benign tremulous parkinsonism. Arch Neurol 63, 354–357

Keus SHJ, Bloem BR, Hendriks EJM, Bredero-Cohen AB, Munneke M (2007): Evidence-based analysis of physical therapy in Parkinson's disease with recommendations for practice and research. Mov Disord 22, 451-460

Khorkova O, Wahlestedt C (2017): Oligonucleotide therapies for disorders of the nervous system. Nat Biotechnol 35, 249–263

Kilpatrick BS (2016): Connecting Ca2+ and lysosomes to Parkinson disease. Messenger (Los Angel) 5, 76–86

Kitada T, Asakawa S, Hattori N, Matsumine H, Yamamura Y, Minoshima S, Yokochi M, Mizuno Y, Shimizu N (1998): Mutations in the parkin gene cause autosomal recessive juvenile parkinsonism. Nature 392, 605-608

Klein C, Westenberger A (2012): Genetics of Parkinson's disease. Cold Spring Harb Perspect Med 2, a008888

Klein ME, Lioy DT, Ma L, Impey S, Mandel G, Goodman RH (2007): Homeostatic regulation of MeCP2 expression by a CREB-induced microRNA. Nat Neurosci 10, 1513–1514

Knöferle J, Ramljak S, Koch JC, Tönges L, Asif AR, Michel U, Wouters FS, Heermann S, Krieglstein K, Zerr I et al. (2010): TGF-beta 1 enhances neurite outgrowth via regulation of proteasome function and EFABP. Neurobiol Dis 38, 395–404

Koch JC, Tönges L, Barski E, Michel U, Bähr M, Lingor P (2014): ROCK2 is a major regulator of axonal degeneration, neuronal death and axonal regeneration in the CNS. Cell Death Dis 5, e1225

Koch JC, Tatenhorst L, Roser A-E, Saal K-A, Tönges L, Lingor P (2018): ROCK inhibition in models of neurodegeneration and its potential for clinical translation. Pharmacol Ther 189, 1–21

Kopin IJ (1992): Features of the dopaminergic neurotoxin MPTP. Ann N Y Acad Sci 648, 96–104

Lambert J-P, Ivosev G, Couzens AL, Larsen B, Taipale M, Lin Z-Y, Zhong Q, Lindquist S, Vidal M, Aebersold R et al. (2013): Mapping differential interactomes by affinity purification coupled with data-independent mass spectrometry acquisition. Nat Methods 10, 1239–1245

Langston JW, Ballard P, Tetrud JW, Irwin I (1983): Chronic Parkinsonism in humans due to a product of meperidine-analog synthesis. Science 219, 979–980

Lau P, Bossers K, Janky R's, Salta E, Frigerio CS, Barbash S, Rothman R, Sierksma ASR, Thathiah A, Greenberg D et al. (2013): Alteration of the microRNA network during the progression of Alzheimer's disease. EMBO Mol Med 5, 1613–1634

Lee A, Gilbert RM (2016): Epidemiology of Parkinson Disease. Neurol Clin 34, 955–965

Lee RC, Feinbaum RL, Ambros V (1993): The C. elegans heterochronic gene lin-4 encodes small RNAs with antisense complementarity to lin-14. Cell 75, 843–854

Lees AJ, Hardy J, Revesz T (2009): Parkinson's disease. Lancet 373, 2055–2066

Leggio L, Vivarelli S, L'Episcopo F, Tirolo C, Caniglia S, Testa N, Marchetti B, Iraci N (2017): microRNAs in Parkinson's Disease: From Pathogenesis to Novel Diagnostic and Therapeutic Approaches. Int J Mol Sci 18, 2698

Lei Z, van Mil A, Brandt MM, Grundmann S, Hoefer I, Smits M, El Azzouzi H, Fukao T, Cheng C, Doevendans PA et al. (2015): MicroRNA-132/212 family enhances arteriogenesis after hindlimb ischaemia through modulation of the Ras-MAPK pathway. J Cell Mol Med 19, 1994–2005

Lill CM (2016): Genetics of Parkinson's disease. Mol Cell Probes 30, 386–396

Lim K-L (2007): Ubiquitin-proteasome system dysfunction in Parkinson's disease: current evidence and controversies. Expert Rev Proteomics 4, 769–781

Lingor P, Unsicker K, Krieglstein K (1999): Midbrain dopaminergic neurons are protected from radical induced damage by GDF-5 application. Short communication. J Neural Transm (Vienna) 106, 139–144

Lingor P, Teusch N, Schwarz K, Mueller R, Mack H, Bähr M, Mueller BK (2007): Inhibition of Rho kinase (ROCK) increases neurite outgrowth on chondroitin sulphate proteoglycan in vitro and axonal regeneration in the adult optic nerve in vivo. J Neurochem 103, 181–189

Lingor P, Carboni E, Koch JC (2017): Alpha-synuclein and iron: Two keys unlocking Parkinson's disease. J Neural Transm (Vienna) 124, 973–981

Lin M-Y, Lin Y-M, Kao T-c, Chuang H-H, Chen R-H (2011): PDZ-RhoGEF ubiquitination by Cullin3-KLHL20 controls neurotrophin-induced neurite outgrowth. J Cell Biol 193, 985–994

Li S, Lv X, Zhai K, Xu R, Zhang Y, Zhao S, Qin X, Yin L, Lou J (2016): MicroRNA-7 inhibits neuronal apoptosis in a cellular Parkinson's disease model by targeting Bax and Sirt2. Am J Transl Res 8, 993–1004

Liu B, Fang F, Pedersen NL, Tillander A, Ludvigsson JF, Ekbom A, Svenningsson P, Chen H, Wirdefeldt K (2017): Vagotomy and Parkinson disease: A Swedish register-based matched-cohort study. Neurology 88, 1996–2002

Li Z, Dong X, Dong X, Wang Z, Liu W, Deng N, Ding Y, Tang L, Hla T, Zeng R et al. (2005): Regulation of PTEN by Rho small GTPases. Nat Cell Biol 7, 399–404

Losensky G, Jung K, Urlaub H, Pfeifer F, Fröls S, Lenz C (2017): Shedding light on biofilm formation of Halobacterium salinarum R1 by SWATH-LC/MS/MS analysis of planktonic and sessile cells. Proteomics 17, 1600111

Lou X, Liao W (2012): Association of Nurr1 gene mutations with Parkinson's disease in the Han population living in the Hubei province of China. Neural Regen Res 7, 1791–1796

Ludwig C, Gillet L, Rosenberger G, Amon S, Collins BC, Aebersold R (2018): Data-independent acquisition-based SWATH-MS for quantitative proteomics: a tutorial. Mol Syst Biol 14, e8126

Luk KC, Kehm VM, Zhang B, O'Brien P, Trojanowski JQ, Lee VMY (2012): Intracerebral inoculation of pathological α-synuclein initiates a rapidly progressive neurodegenerative α-synucleinopathy in mice. J Exp Med 209, 975–986

Lunenfeld B, Stratton P (2013): The clinical consequences of an ageing world and preventive strategies. Best Pract Res Clin Obstet Gynaecol 27, 643–659

Luo J, Meng C, Tang Y, Zhang S, Wan M, Bi Y, Zhou X (2014): miR-132/212 cluster inhibits the growth of lung cancer xenografts in nude mice. Int J Clin Exp Med 7, 4115–4122

Luo L (2000): Rho GTPases in neuronal morphogenesis. Nat Rev Neurosci 1, 173–180

Magill ST, Cambronne XA, Luikart BW, Lioy DT, Leighton BH, Westbrook GL, Mandel G, Goodman RH (2010): microRNA-132 regulates dendritic growth and arborization of newborn neurons in the adult hippocampus. Proc Natl Acad Sci U S A 107, 20382–20387

Mann VM, Cooper JM, Daniel SE, Srai K, Jenner P, Marsden CD, Schapira AH (1994): Complex I, iron, and ferritin in Parkinson's disease substantia nigra. Ann Neurol 36, 876–881

Marmor-Kollet N, Schuldiner O (2016): Contrasting developmental axon regrowth and neurite sprouting of Drosophila mushroom body neurons reveals shared and unique molecular mechanisms. Dev Neurobiol 76, 262–276

Marques TM, Kuiperij HB, Bruinsma IB, van Rumund A, Aerts MB, Esselink RAJ, Bloem BR, Verbeek MM (2017): MicroRNAs in Cerebrospinal Fluid as Potential Biomarkers for Parkinson's Disease and Multiple System Atrophy. Mol Neurobiol 54, 7736–7745

Martin-Bastida A, Ward RJ, Newbould R, Piccini P, Sharp D, Kabba C, Patel MC, Spino M, Connelly J, Tricta F et al. (2017): Brain iron chelation by deferiprone in a phase 2 randomised double-blinded placebo controlled clinical trial in Parkinson's disease. Sci Rep 7, 1398

Massano J, Bhatia KP (2012): Clinical approach to Parkinson's disease: features, diagnosis, and principles of management. Cold Spring Harb Perspect Med 2, a008870

Matsukawa T, Morita K, Omizu S, Kato S, Koriyama Y (2018): Mechanisms of RhoA inactivation and CDC42 and Rac1 activation during zebrafish optic nerve regeneration. Neurochem Int 112, 71–80

McFarland KN, Huizenga MN, Darnell SB, Sangrey GR, Berezovska O, Cha J-HJ, Outeiro TF, Sadri-Vakili G (2014): MeCP2: A novel Huntingtin interactor. Hum Mol Genet 23, 1036–1044

Mehta A, Zhao JL, Sinha N, Marinov GK, Mann M, Kowalczyk MS, Galimidi RP, Du X, Erikci E, Regev A et al. (2015): The MicroRNA-132 and MicroRNA-212 Cluster Regulates Hematopoietic Stem Cell Maintenance and Survival with Age by Buffering FOXO3 Expression. Immunity 42, 1021–1032

Mendoza-Viveros L, Chiang C-K, Ong JLK, Hegazi S, Cheng AH, Bouchard-Cannon P, Fana M, Lowden C, Zhang P, Bothorel B et al. (2017): miR-132/212 Modulates Seasonal Adaptation and Dendritic Morphology of the Central Circadian Clock. Cell Rep 19, 505–520

Mhyre TR, Boyd JT, Hamill RW, Maguire-Zeiss KA (2012): Parkinson's disease. Subcell Biochem 65, 389–455

Miller DB, O'Callaghan JP (2015): Biomarkers of Parkinson's disease: Present and future. Metab Clin Exp 64, 40-46

Mitra K, Gangopadhaya PK, Das SK (2003): Parkinsonism plus syndrome--a review. Neurol India 51, 183–188

Miyazaki I, Asanuma M (2008): Dopaminergic neuron-specific oxidative stress caused by dopamine itself. Acta Med Okayama 62, 141–150

Mizuki Y, Takaki M, Sakamoto S, Okamoto S, Kishimoto M, Okahisa Y, Itoh M, Yamada N (2016): Human Rho Guanine Nucleotide Exchange Factor 11 (ARHGEF11) Regulates Dendritic Morphogenesis. Int J Mol Sci 18, 67

Moldovan A-S, Groiss SJ, Elben S, Sudmeyer M, Schnitzler A, Wojtecki L (2015): The treatment of Parkinson's disease with deep brain stimulation: current issues. Neural Regen Res 10, 1018–1022

Moon SY, Zang H, Zheng Y (2003): Characterization of a brain-specific Rho GTPase-activating protein, p200RhoGAP. J Biol Chem 278, 4151–4159

Moore DJ, Dawson VL, Dawson TM (2003): Role for the Ubiquitin-Proteasome System in Parkinson's Disease and Other Neurodegenerative Brain Amyloidoses. Neuromolecular Med 4, 95–108

Nakayama AY, Harms MB, Luo L (2000): Small GTPases Rac and Rho in the maintenance of dendritic spines and branches in hippocampal pyramidal neurons. J Neurosci 20, 5329–5338

Nakazawa T, Watabe AM, Tezuka T, Yoshida Y, Yokoyama K, Umemori H, Inoue A, Okabe S, Manabe T, Yamamoto T (2003): p250GAP, a novel brain-enriched GTPase-activating protein for Rho family GTPases, is involved in the N-methyl-d-aspartate receptor signaling. Mol Biol Cell 14, 2921–2934

Niccoli T, Partridge L (2012): Ageing as a risk factor for disease. Curr Biol 22, 741-752

Nuytemans K, Theuns J, Cruts M, van Broeckhoven C (2010): Genetic etiology of Parkinson disease associated with mutations in the SNCA, PARK2, PINK1, PARK7, and LRRK2 genes: a mutation update. Hum Mutat 31, 763–780

Oertel W, Schulz JB (2016): Current and experimental treatments of Parkinson disease: A guide for neuroscientists. J Neurochem 139 Suppl 1, 325–337

Oertel W, Müller H, Schade-Brittinger C, Kamp C, Balthasar K, Articus K, Brinkman M, Venuto C, Unger M, Eggert K et al. (2018): The NIC-PD-study – A randomized, placebo-controlled, double-blind, multi-centre trial to assess the disease-modifying potential of transdermal nicotine in early Parkinson's disease in Germany and N. America. https://www.mdsabstracts.org/abstract/the-nic-pd-study-a-randomized-placebo-controlled-double-blind-multi-centre-trial-to-assess-the-disease-modifying-potential-of-transdermal-nicotine-in-early-parkinsons-disease-in-g/, accessed 16.07.2019

Ohtake Y, Hayat U, Li S (2015): PTEN inhibition and axon regeneration and neural repair. Neural Regen Res 10, 1363–1368

Okabe T, Nakamura T, Nishimura YN, Kohu K, Ohwada S, Morishita Y, Akiyama T (2003): RICS, a novel GTPase-activating protein for Cdc42 and Rac1, is involved in the beta-catenin-N-cadherin and N-methyl-D-aspartate receptor signaling. J Biol Chem 278, 9920–9927

Olanow CW, Goetz CG, Kordower JH, Stoessl AJ, Sossi V, Brin MF, Shannon KM, Nauert GM, Perl DP, Godbold J et al. (2003): A double-blind controlled trial of bilateral fetal nigral transplantation in Parkinson's disease. Ann Neurol 54, 403–414

Olanow CW, Kieburtz K, Odin P, Espay AJ, Standaert DG, Fernandez HH, Vanagunas A, Othman AA, Widnell KL, Robieson WZ et al. (2014): Continuous intrajejunal infusion of levodopa-carbidopa intestinal gel for patients with advanced Parkinson's disease: A randomised, controlled, double-blind, double-dummy study. Lancet Neurol 13, 141–149

Oliveros JC (2007): VENNY. An interactive tool for comparing lists with Venn Diagrams. https://bioinfogp.cnb.csic.es/tools/venny/, accessed 01.09.2019

Outeiro TF, Kontopoulos E, Altmann SM, Kufareva I, Strathearn KE, Amore AM, Volk CB, Maxwell MM, Rochet J-C, McLean PJ et al. (2007): Sirtuin 2 inhibitors rescue alpha-synuclein-mediated toxicity in models of Parkinson's disease. Science 317, 516–519

Parkinson J (2002): An essay on the shaking palsy. 1817. J Neuropsychiatry Clin Neurosci 14, 223-236

Park J-K, Henry JC, Jiang J, Esau C, Gusev Y, Lerner MR, Postier RG, Brackett DJ, Schmittgen TD (2011): miR-132 and miR-212 are increased in pancreatic cancer and target the retinoblastoma tumor suppressor. Biochem Biophys Res Commun 406, 518–523

Park J-S, Davis RL, Sue CM (2018): Mitochondrial Dysfunction in Parkinson's Disease: New Mechanistic Insights and Therapeutic Perspectives. Curr Neurol Neurosci Rep 18, 21

Parkkinen L, O'Sullivan SS, Collins C, Petrie A, Holton JL, Revesz T, Lees AJ (2011): Disentangling the relationship between lewy bodies and nigral neuronal loss in Parkinson's disease. J Parkinsons Dis 1, 277–286

Park KK, Liu K, Hu Y, Smith PD, Wang C, Cai B, Xu B, Connolly L, Kramvis I, Sahin M et al. (2008): Promoting axon regeneration in the adult CNS by modulation of the PTEN/mTOR pathway. Science 322, 963–966

Pathania M, Torres-Reveron J, Yan L, Kimura T, Lin TV, Gordon V, Teng Z-Q, Zhao X, Fulga TA, van Vactor D et al. (2012): miR-132 enhances dendritic morphogenesis, spine density, synaptic integration, and survival of newborn olfactory bulb neurons. PLoS One 7, e38174

Polymeropoulos MH, Lavedan C, Leroy E, Ide SE, Dehejia A, Dutra A, Pike B, Root H, Rubenstein J, Boyer R et al. (1997): Mutation in the alpha-synuclein gene identified in families with Parkinson's disease. Science 276, 2045–2047

Postuma RB, Berg D, Stern M, Poewe W, Olanow CW, Oertel W, Obeso J, Marek K, Litvan I, Lang AE et al. (2015a): MDS clinical diagnostic criteria for Parkinson's disease. Mov Disord 30, 1591–1601

Postuma RB, Gagnon J-F, Bertrand J-A, Génier Marchand D, Montplaisir JY (2015b): Parkinson risk in idiopathic REM sleep behavior disorder: Preparing for neuroprotective trials. Neurology 84, 1104–1113

Postuma RB, Anang J, Pelletier A, Joseph L, Moscovich M, Grimes D, Furtado S, Munhoz RP, Appel-Cresswell S, Moro A et al. (2017): Caffeine as symptomatic treatment for Parkinson disease (Café-PD): A randomized trial. Neurology 89, 1795–1803

Postuma RB, Poewe W, Litvan I, Lewis S, Lang AE, Halliday G, Goetz CG, Chan P, Slow E, Seppi K et al. (2018): Validation of the MDS clinical diagnostic criteria for Parkinson's disease. Mov Disord 33, 1601–1608

Puspita L, Chung SY, Shim J-W (2017): Oxidative stress and cellular pathologies in Parkinson's disease. Mol Brain 10, 53

Remenyi J, Hunter CJ, Cole C, Ando H, Impey S, Monk CE, Martin KJ, Barton GJ, Hutvagner G, Arthur JSC (2010): Regulation of the miR-212/132 locus by MSK1 and CREB in response to neurotrophins. Biochem J 428, 281–291

Riggs AD, Porter TN (1996): Overview of epigenetic mechanisms. Cold Spring Harbor Monograph Archive 32, 29–45

Ritz B, Lee P-C, Lassen CF, Arah OA (2014): Parkinson disease and smoking revisited: ease of quitting is an early sign of the disease. Neurology 83, 1396–1402

Roser AE: miRNAs in protection and regeneration of dopaminergic midbrain neurons. book (rer. nat.). Göttingen 2016

Roser AE, Caldi Gomes L, Schünemann J, Maass F, Lingor P (2018a): Circulating miRNAs as Diagnostic Biomarkers for Parkinson's Disease. Front Neurosci 12, 625

Roser AE, Caldi Gomes L, Halder R, Jain G, Maass F, Tönges L, Tatenhorst L, Bähr M, Fischer A, Lingor P (2018b): miR-182-5p and miR-183-5p Act as GDNF Mimics in Dopaminergic Midbrain Neurons. Mol Ther Nucleic Acids 11, 9–22

Rupaimoole R, Slack FJ (2017): MicroRNA therapeutics: towards a new era for the management of cancer and other diseases. Nature Reviews Drug Discovery 16, 203-222

Ryan BJ, Hoek S, Fon EA, Wade-Martins R (2015): Mitochondrial dysfunction and mitophagy in Parkinson's: from familial to sporadic disease. Trends Biochem Sci 40, 200–210

Saal K-A, Koch JC, Tatenhorst L, Szego EM, Ribas VT, Michel U, Bahr M, Tonges L, Lingor P (2015): AAV.shRNA-mediated downregulation of ROCK2 attenuates degeneration of dopaminergic neurons in toxin-induced models of Parkinson's disease in vitro and in vivo. Neurobiol Dis 73, 150–162

Sai X, Yonemura S, Ladher RK (2014): Junctionally restricted RhoA activity is necessary for apical constriction during phase 2 inner ear placode invagination. Dev Biol 394, 206–216

Sampathu DM, Giasson BI, Pawlyk AC, Trojanowski JQ, Lee VM-Y (2003): Ubiquitination of α-Synuclein Is Not Required for Formation of Pathological Inclusions in α-Synucleinopathies. Am J Pathol 163, 91–100

Santo EE, Stroeken P, Sluis PV, Koster J, Versteeg R, Westerhout EM (2013): FOXO3a is a major target of inactivation by PI3K/AKT signaling in aggressive neuroblastoma. Cancer Res 73, 2189–2198

Savica R, Grossardt BR, Bower JH, Ahlskog JE, Rocca WA (2016): Time Trends in the Incidence of Parkinson Disease. JAMA Neurol 73, 981–989

Schapira AH, Mann VM, Cooper JM, Dexter D, Daniel SE, Jenner P, Clark JB, Marsden CD (1990): Anatomic and disease specificity of NADH CoQ1 reductase (complex I) deficiency in Parkinson's disease. J Neurochem 55, 2142–2145

Scheperjans F, Aho V, Pereira PAB, Koskinen K, Paulin L, Pekkonen E, Haapaniemi E, Kaakkola S, Eerola-Rautio J, Pohja M et al. (2015): Gut microbiota are related to Parkinson's disease and clinical phenotype. Mov Disord 30, 350–358

Schwarzschild MA, Ascherio A, Beal MF, Cudkowicz ME, Curhan GC, Hare JM, Hooper DC, Kieburtz KD, Macklin EA, Oakes D et al. (2014): Inosine to increase serum and cerebrospinal fluid urate in Parkinson disease: A randomized clinical trial. JAMA Neurol 71, 141–150

Scoto M, Finkel R, Mercuri E, Muntoni F (2018): Genetic therapies for inherited neuromuscular disorders. Lancet Child Adolesc Health 2, 600–609

Selikhova M, Williams DR, Kempster PA, Holton JL, Revesz T, Lees AJ (2009): A clinicopathological study of subtypes in Parkinson's disease. Brain 132, 2947–2957

Shin H-W, Chung SJ (2012): Drug-induced parkinsonism. J Clin Neurol 8, 15–21

Siomi H, Siomi MC (2009): On the road to reading the RNA-interference code. Nature 457, 396–404

Smith PY, Hernandez-Rapp J, Jolivette F, Lecours C, Bisht K, Goupil C, Dorval V, Parsi S, Morin F, Planel E et al. (2015): miR-132/212 deficiency impairs tau metabolism and promotes pathological aggregation in vivo. Hum Mol Genet 24, 6721–6735

Smythies J, Edelstein L, Ramachandran V (2014): Molecular mechanisms for the inheritance of acquired characteristics-exosomes, microRNA shuttling, fear and stress: Lamarck resurrected? Front Genet 5, 133

Song G, Wang L (2008): MiR-433 and miR-127 arise from independent overlapping primary transcripts encoded by the miR-433-127 locus. PLoS One 3, e3574

Spillantini MG, Schmidt ML, Lee VMY, Trojanowski JQ, Jakes R, Goedert M (1997): α-Synuclein in Lewy bodies. Nature 388, 839-840

Stefanis L (2012): alpha-Synuclein in Parkinson's disease. Cold Spring Harb Perspect Med 2, a009399

Stoicea N, Du A, Lakis DC, Tipton C, Arias-Morales CE, Bergese SD (2016): The MiRNA Journey from Theory to Practice as a CNS Biomarker. Front Genet 7, 11

Sun S, Han X, Li X, Song Q, Lu M, Jia M, Ding J, Hu G (2018): MicroRNA-212-5p Prevents Dopaminergic Neuron Death by Inhibiting SIRT2 in MPTP-Induced Mouse Model of Parkinson's Disease. Front Mol Neurosci 11, 381

Sun SM, Rockova V, Bullinger L, Dijkstra MK, Döhner H, Löwenberg B, Jongen-Lavrencic M (2013): The prognostic relevance of miR-212 expression with survival in cytogenetically and molecularly heterogeneous AML. Leukemia 27, 100

Svensson E, Horvath-Puho E, Thomsen RW, Djurhuus JC, Pedersen L, Borghammer P, Sorensen HT (2015): Vagotomy and subsequent risk of Parkinson's disease. Ann Neurol 78, 522–529

Tagliaferro P, Burke RE (2016): Retrograde Axonal Degeneration in Parkinson Disease. J Parkinsons Dis 6, 1–15

Thenganatt MA, Jankovic J (2014): Parkinson disease subtypes. JAMA Neurol 71, 499–504

Thum T, Chowdhury K, Ucar A, Gupta SK (2013): The mirna-212/132 family as a therapeutic target. https://patents.google.com/patent/WO2013034653A1/en, accessed 01.09.2019

Titze-de-Almeida R, Titze-de-Almeida SS (2018): miR-7 Replacement Therapy in Parkinson's Disease. Curr Gene Ther 18, 143–153

Tolosa E, Wenning G, Poewe W (2006): The diagnosis of Parkinson's disease. Lancet Neurology 5, 75–86

Tompkins MM, Hill WD (1997): Contribution of somal Lewy bodies to neuronal death. Brain Res 775, 24–29

Tonges L, Planchamp V, Koch J-C, Herdegen T, Bahr M, Lingor P (2011): JNK isoforms differentially regulate neurite growth and regeneration in dopaminergic neurons in vitro. J Mol Neurosci 45, 284–293

Tufekci KU, Meuwissen R, Genc S, Genc K (2012): Inflammation in Parkinson's disease. Adv Protein Chem Struct Biol 88, 69–132

Tyanova S, Temu T, Sinitcyn P, Carlson A, Hein MY, Geiger T, Mann M, Cox J (2016): The Perseus computational platform for comprehensive analysis of (prote)omics data. Nat Methods 13, 731–740

Tysnes O-B, Storstein A (2017): Epidemiology of Parkinson's disease. J Neural Transm (Vienna) 124, 901–905

Ucar A, Gupta SK, Fiedler J, Erikci E, Kardasinski M, Batkai S, Dangwal S, Kumarswamy R, Bang C, Holzmann A et al. (2012): The miRNA-212/132 family regulates both cardiac hypertrophy and cardiomyocyte autophagy. Nat Commun 3, 1078

Venter JC, Adams MD, Myers EW, Li PW, Mural RJ, Sutton GG, Smith HO, Yandell M, Evans CA, Holt RA et al. (2001): The sequence of the human genome. Science 291, 1304–1351

Vo N, Klein ME, Varlamova O, Keller DM, Yamamoto T, Goodman RH, Impey S (2005): A cAMP-response element binding protein-induced microRNA regulates neuronal morphogenesis. Proc Natl Acad Sci U S A 102, 16426–16431

Wada R, Akiyama Y, Hashimoto Y, Fukamachi H, Yuasa Y (2010): miR-212 is downregulated and suppresses methyl-CpG-binding protein MeCP2 in human gastric cancer. Int J Cancer 127, 1106–1114

Waddington CH (2012): The epigenotype. 1942. Int J Epidemiol 41, 10–13

Wahl S, Barth H, Ciossek T, Aktories K, Mueller BK (2000): Ephrin-A5 induces collapse of growth cones by activating Rho and Rho kinase. J Cell Biol 149, 263–270

Wakabayashi K, Takahashi H, Takeda S, Ohama E, Ikuta F (1988): Parkinson's disease: The presence of Lewy bodies in Auerbach's and Meissner's plexuses. Acta Neuropathol 76, 217–221

Wanet A, Tacheny A, Arnould T, Renard P (2012): miR-212/132 expression and functions: within and beyond the neuronal compartment. Nucleic Acids Res 40, 4742–4753

Wang F, Wang J, Ju L, Chen L, Cai W, Yang J (2018a): Diagnostic and prognostic potential of serum miR-132/212 cluster in patients with hepatocellular carcinoma. Ann Clin Biochem, 576-582

Wang H, Duan X, Ren Y, Liu Y, Huang M, Liu P, Wang R, Gao G, Zhou L, Feng Z et al. (2013a): FoxO3a Negatively Regulates Nerve Growth Factor-Induced Neuronal Differentiation Through Inhibiting the Expression of Neurochondrin in PC12 Cells. Mol Neurobiol 47, 24–36

Wang T, Li B, Yuan X, Cui L, Wang Z, Zhang Y, Yu M, Xiu Y, Zhang Z, Li W et al. (2018b): MiR-20a Plays a Key Regulatory Role in the Repair of Spinal Cord Dorsal Column Lesion via PDZ-RhoGEF/RhoA/GAP43 Axis in Rat. Cell Mol Neurobiol 39, 87–98

Wang X (2014): Composition of seed sequence is a major determinant of microRNA targeting patterns. Bioinformatics 30, 1377–1383

Wang Z, Yao H, Lin S, Zhu X, Shen Z, Lu G, Poon WS, Xie D, Lin MC, Kung H (2013b): Transcriptional and epigenetic regulation of human microRNAs. Cancer Lett 331, 1–10

Wayman GA, Davare M, Ando H, Fortin D, Varlamova O, Cheng H-YM, Marks D, Obrietan K, Soderling TR, Goodman RH et al. (2008): An activity-regulated microRNA controls dendritic plasticity by down-regulating p250GAP. Proc Natl Acad Sci U S A 105, 9093–9098

Westbrook TF, Hu G, Ang XL, Mulligan P, Pavlova NN, Liang A, Leng Y, Maehr R, Shi Y, Harper JW et al. (2008): SCFbeta-TRCP controls oncogenic transformation and neural differentiation through REST degradation. Nature 452, 370–374

Winter J, Jung S, Keller S, Gregory RI, Diederichs S (2009): Many roads to maturity: microRNA biogenesis pathways and their regulation. Nat Cell Biol 11, 228–234

Wong H-KA, Veremeyko T, Patel N, Lemere CA, Walsh DM, Esau C, Vanderburg C, Krichevsky AM (2013): De-repression of FOXO3a death axis by microRNA-132 and -212 causes neuronal apoptosis in Alzheimer's disease. Hum Mol Genet 22, 3077–3092

Yang D, Li T, Wang Y, Tang Y, Cui H, Tang Y, Zhang X, Chen D, Shen N, Le W (2012): miR-132 regulates the differentiation of dopamine neurons by directly targeting Nurr1 expression. J Cell Sci 125, 1673–1682

Yan MH, Wang X, Zhu X (2013): Mitochondrial defects and oxidative stress in Alzheimer disease and Parkinson disease. Free Radic Biol Med 62, 90–101

Zecca L, Youdim MBH, Riederer P, Connor JR, Crichton RR (2004): Iron, brain ageing and neurodegenerative disorders. Nature Reviews Neuroscience 5, 863-873

Zesiewicz TA, Kuo S-H (2015): Essential tremor. BMJ Clin Evid 2015, 1206

Zhang P-L, Chen Y, Zhang C-H, Wang Y-X, Fernandez-Funez P (2018): Genetics of Parkinson's disease and related disorders. J Med Genet 55, 73–80

Zhang S, Hao J, Xie F, Hu X, Liu C, Tong J, Zhou J, Wu J, Shao C (2011): Downregulation of miR-132 by promoter methylation contributes to pancreatic cancer development. Carcinogenesis 32, 1183–1189

Zhang Y, Bilbao A, Bruderer T, Luban J, Strambio-De-Castillia C, Lisacek F, Hopfgartner G, Varesio E (2015): The Use of Variable Q1 Isolation Windows Improves Selectivity in LC-SWATH-MS Acquisition. J Proteome Res 14, 4359–4371

Zhao C, Ma H, Bossy-Wetzel E, Lipton SA, Zhang Z, Feng G-S (2003): GC-GAP, a Rho family GTPase-activating protein that interacts with signaling adapters Gab1 and Gab2. J Biol Chem 278, 34641–34653

Zhao Y, Zhao R, Wu J, Wang Q, Pang K, Shi Q, Gao Q, Hu Y, Dong X, Zhang J et al. (2018): Melatonin protects against Aβ-induced neurotoxicity· in primary neurons via miR-132/PTEN/AKT/FOXO3a pathway. Biofactors 44, 609–618

Zocchi L, Sassone-Corsi P (2012): SIRT1-mediated deacetylation of MeCP2 contributes to BDNF expression. Epigenetics 7, 695–700

Zuo YC, Li HL, Xiong NX, Shen JY, Huang YZ, Fu P, Zhao HY (2016): Overexpression of Tau Rescues Nogo-66-Induced Neurite Outgrowth Inhibition In Vitro. Neurosci Bull 32, 577–584

www.ingramcontent.com/pod-product-compliance
Lightning Source LLC
LaVergne TN
LVHW041125150826
845673LV00007B/2184

* 9 7 8 3 3 8 4 2 5 4 6 5 8 *